Eating Together

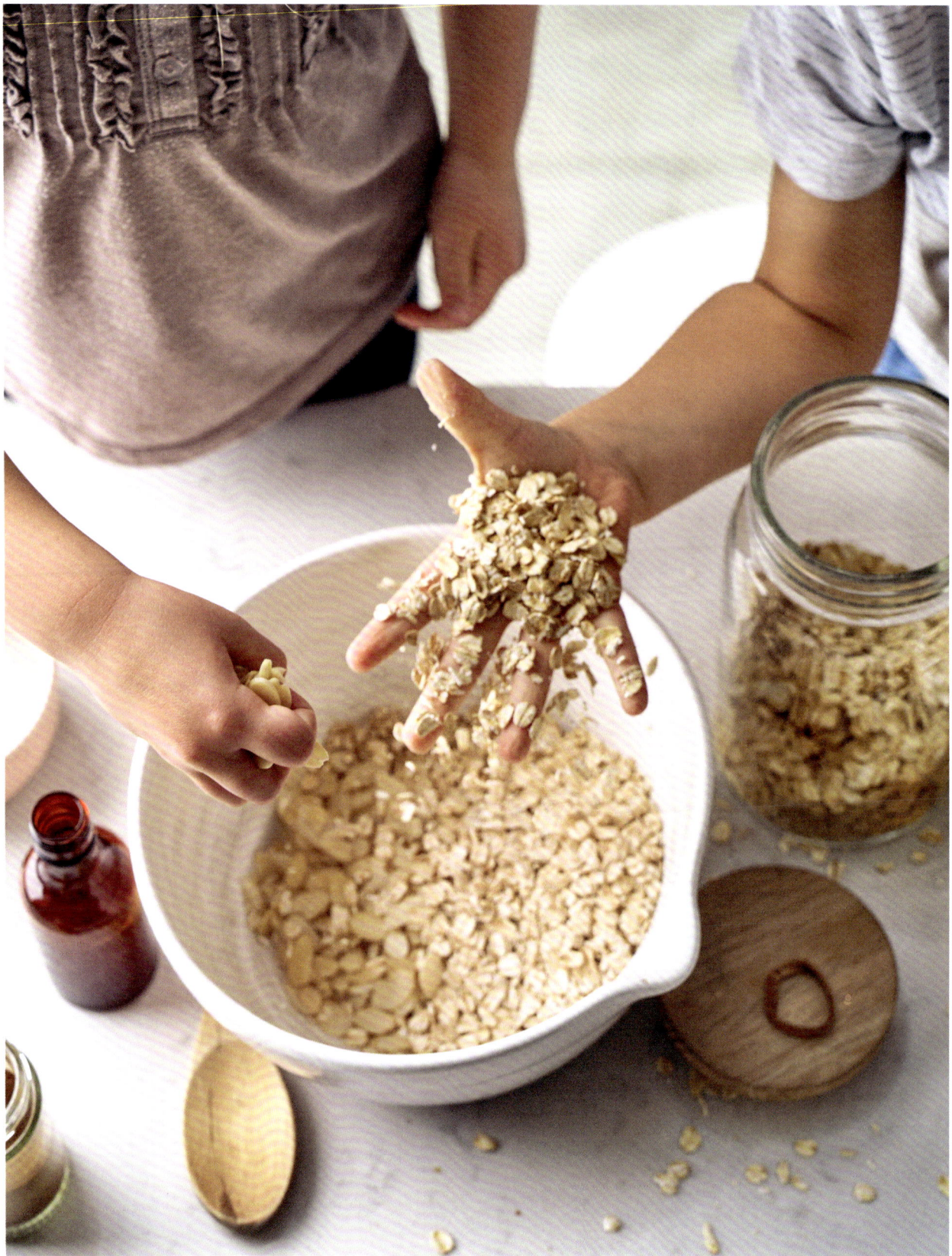

Eating Together

A recipe for healthier, happier families

DR CLARE BAILEY MOSLEY
& PROFESSOR STEPHEN SCOTT

℃ℬ

*For Michael, the children and those wonderful years
of eating together – Clare*

*For Penny, Ed, Jonny and Adam for the good times spent
enjoying each other's company around the table – Stephen*

First published in Great Britain in 2025
by Short Books, an imprint of
Octopus Publishing Group Ltd
Carmelite House
50 Victoria Embankment
London EC4Y 0DZ
www.octopusbooks.co.uk
www.octopusbooksusa.com

An Hachette UK Company
www.hachette.co.uk

The authorized representative in the EEA is
Hachette Ireland, 8 Castlecourt Centre, Dublin
15, D15 XTP3, Ireland (email: info@hbgi.ie)

Text copyright © Dr Clare Bailey Mosley
and Professor Stephen Scott 2025

All recipes written by Dr Clare Bailey Mosley
and Kathryn Bruton.

Distributed in the US by Hachette Book Group,
1290 Avenue of the Americas, 4th and 5th
Floors, New York, NY 10104

Distributed in Canada by Canadian Manda
Group, 664 Annette St, Toronto, Ontario,
Canada M6S 2C8

ISBN: 9781780725840
eISBN: 9781780725857

A CIP catalogue record for this book is available
from the British Library.

Printed and bound in China.

10 9 8 7 6 5 4 3 2 1

Publisher: Jo Morrell
Art Director: Yasia Williams
Designer: Lizzie Ballantyne
Senior Editor: Leanne Bryan
Copy Editor: Jo Roberts-Miller
Photographer: Kate Whitaker
Food Stylist: Becks Wilkinson
Props Stylist: Hannah Wilkinson
Illustrator: David Gifford
Senior Production Manager: Katherine Hockley

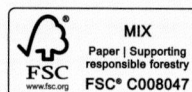

FSC
www.fsc.org

MIX
Paper | Supporting
responsible forestry
FSC® C008047

Contents

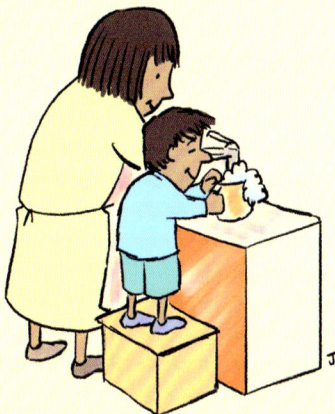

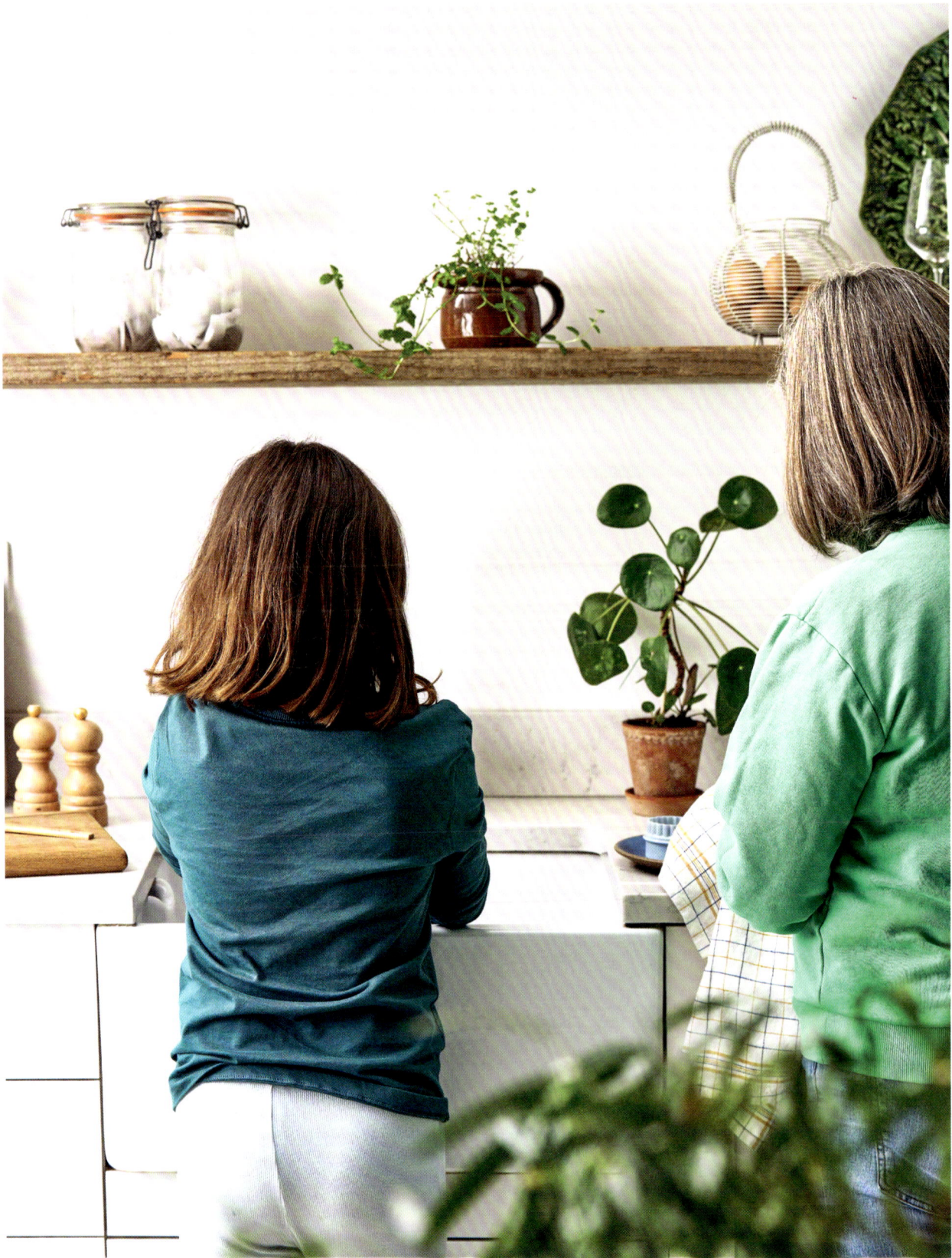

Preface by Professor Stephen Scott

Stephen Scott is Professor of Child Health and Behaviour at the Institute of Psychiatry, Psychology and Neuroscience at King's College London; and Consultant Child and Adolescent Psychiatrist at the Maudsley Hospital

It has always fascinated me that, despite a full degree in psychology followed by medical studies at Cambridge and five years working in paediatrics at Great Ormond Street Hospital, when I became a father, I couldn't stop my three-day-old son screaming his head off. Over time (and having seen three sons through to adulthood), I became more and more interested in understanding the ways parents' behaviour affects their children.

I was fortunate to be appointed head of the parenting clinic at the Maudsley Hospital, where for the last 30 years we have been working with families to research and test the most effective ways parents can help their children become happier and better adjusted, as well as becoming better readers, faster learners and having improved brain growth.

Clare and I got to know each other originally because her mother, Veira Bailey, was a child psychiatrist like me and our paths crossed many times. With a background in medicine and four children of her own, Clare was always fascinated by parenting and we worked together to develop an evidence-based online parenting programme called Parenting Matters, which is centred on a concept we called 'LOVE and LIMITS'. In Clare I met someone who was passionate about disseminating that information in such a way that all parents – regardless of income, background, personality and parenting style – could create better bonds with their children and be better placed to set their children up to be balanced, inquisitive and interested young people. We worked together to bring parenting workshops to schools and corporations. Then, just before lockdown, we went live with our www.parentingmatters.co.uk online programme. It was a great collaborative effort and was well received.

We started talking about writing a parenting book together and, with Clare's late husband Michael Mosley, we developed the idea that eating together as a family could provide an excellent opportunity to practise beneficial parenting techniques. Michael also believed that making family meals a regular habit could improve nutrition for both parents and children. We rapidly realised that if we focused on Clare's passion for creating healthy and delicious recipes the whole family could enjoy, we might just have stumbled on a winning formula. Michael thought it was a great idea, and it is a great shame he's no longer around to see the proposal come to fruition.

When there is so much scientific evidence to support the hypothesis that eating together as a family can improve the mental and physical health of everyone involved, creating stronger bonds between you and your children that could go on to shape the rest of their lives, why would you not want to give it a try?

Eating together is 'just one thing' of which Michael would, most certainly, have approved.

Preface by Dr Clare Bailey Mosley

Clare Bailey Mosley, wife of Dr Michael Mosley, is a GP and author of several bestselling recipe books. She studied Psychology and combines her work with her passion for supporting parents with their parenting strategies

When I was growing up in the 1960s and 1970s, we always ate our meals together sitting around the table as a family. It was one of the few set fixtures of the day. Whatever we were doing, we were expected to be home in time to help prepare and eat our evening meal. I was one of four children, and from a young age we were each given tasks to help put the meal together, to lay the table and also clear away and wash up afterwards. When Michael and I married and our four children came along, I was determined that the tradition would continue. In the early days, when we were both working, we tended to serve up a lot of fish fingers and chicken nuggets with minimal greens, which kept the kids happy (and Michael, too). Family mealtimes had been a very important part of both our upbringings, and it seemed natural to want to try to repeat that pattern with our own children. We were lucky to have the flexibility with our work that allowed it to happen. Those are such wonderfully warm memories – everyone around the table, laughing, chatting and fighting to get a word in edgeways.

It was only after 2012, when Michael was diagnosed with type 2 diabetes and lost loads of weight on his 5:2 Fast Diet, that I really started getting interested in how to ensure the whole family ate healthily. Helping to create the recipes for Michael's Blood Sugar Diet books in 2016 was play time for me, and I loved it. By then, our four children were beginning to eat more adventurously, and I'd try to get them to help me in the kitchen – preparing food and experimenting with recipes – and they would negotiate the various tidying-up chores between them. I remember Michael often trying to slip away after the meal on the pretext of work to avoid the washing up!

For many of those years I worked as a GP, which gave me a great insight into the challenges many families face. It became clear to me that, as parents, we all do our very best, but we're not working from a guidebook. We muddle along as best we can, facing numerous challenges and shouldering the responsibility of bringing up our children alone. I was keen to hone my own parenting skills, as there is always scope for improvement, and I wanted to enhance my professional training in order to offer support to other parents, too. This is when I chased up my friend Professor Stephen Scott and signed up for his gold-standard training programme in parenting at the Institute of Psychiatry in London. With extra qualifications under my belt, I went on to devise and deliver parenting courses, initially speaking to local parents, then going into large corporations and giving seminars to the parents among their staff. Following that, I put those learnings into an online course, so I could reach and teach a wider audience.

Stephen, Michael and I often talked about the important place family meals take in the parenting mix, and we shared our concerns about the way this lovely ritual has been slowly slipping away. Believe me, I know only too well just how hectic life with young kids can be. The opportunities to sit down together at mealtimes are being squeezed out. When your working day has to fit around distributing children between various after-school clubs, it can be so much easier to heat something up in the microwave than agonise over how many peas each child has managed to eat. But there's growing evidence to suggest that families who cook and eat together are more likely to eat healthily. And, beyond that, there are plenty of studies showing the huge benefits of eating together, and how it provides an important, safe, predictable time for family members to connect, repair relationships and have fun.

Michael and I often discussed my passion for helping parents and he, like me, was convinced that eating together was one simple thing that really benefits family dynamics, at the same time as increasing awareness and consumption of healthy food. So, while I was working to create and test delicious, nutritionally balanced and calorie-counted recipes for his Fast 800 plan, I was quietly accumulating a notebook of family meals, thinking all the time about how children could get involved in food preparation so they could expand their taste repertoires and learn to love good, healthy, home-cooked meals. For adults who are counting calories, the information is on pages 200–3.

Over the years, I've worked closely with food writer Kathryn Bruton to fine-tune the recipes and ensure they always pack a nutritional punch. For this book, she drafted in her young daughters to be tasters and took on board my advice about trying to get the whole family sitting down to regular meals together. Now she says that advice has changed the way her girls like to eat and that eating together has become one of the most important things they do as a family, and truly one of the most joyful.

I'm so excited to be able to share some of our favourite recipes in this book, and to be able to combine them with expert, research-backed advice for how to use mealtimes to better bond with your children, build strong relationships and enhance mental resilience, as well as physical health. The good news is that the benefits start straight away and with every tiny move in the right direction – inviting the kids to put their own toppings on a pizza, asking them to pick a recipe they'd like to try, clearing the table of clutter and making sure there are enough chairs for everyone to sit down, or ear-marking just one special meal when you'll stay at the table after the food is finished and play silly games together (see pages 38–9).

I do hope I've whetted your appetite, and that this book inspires you to make eating together a regular fixture for your family.

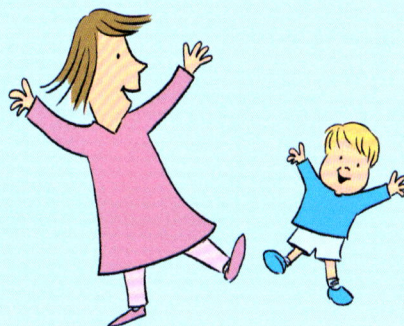

Preface by Dr Clare Bailey Mosley   9

The challenge

Parenting might be one of the most wonderful jobs you ever get to do but, let's be completely honest, it can sometimes feel like a tough and thankless task. Most of us happily take on this role with no training or qualifications, and it is hardly surprising that at times we end up frustrated, or humiliated, when even our best efforts don't seem good enough and we just can't find a way to navigate the tantrums, the misbehaviours and the feeling of overwhelm.

And, no, you're not imagining it. Raising children today really is harder than it ever used to be. We're having to face unique challenges that simply didn't exist in our parents' and grandparents' time. Between the explosion of technology, mounting academic pressures, mental health concerns and social media risks, the landscape has shifted, which means parenting really is more complex and exhausting now than ever.

One big factor is time. Or more precisely, the lack of time. With many parents now working horribly long hours and children tied up with homework (even at a very young age), after-school clubs, hundreds of TV channels, computer games and social media, the opportunities to spend quality time together as a family have rapidly shrunk. We might be trying our hardest to connect with our kids, perhaps trying to supervise every minute detail of their busy lives (helicopter parenting can be exhausting!), but we are all too often battling against the distracting lure of flashing screens and junk food, both of which have been specifically designed to be addictive.

Parents are doing their best but, with so much going on, children don't have the 'free time' we enjoyed as kids. This means they are missing out on valuable opportunities to learn to play independently, to enjoy a sense of complete freedom, make decisions on their own and take (small) risks, to let their minds drift, and to be occasionally bored. But this is how children go on to develop the resilience they need to carry themselves through to adulthood. So many children today are living in a perpetually stimulated state where their rapidly evolving brains are constantly bombarded with information and all their activities are closely monitored. This goes a long way to explain why so many children are experiencing escalating levels of anxiety.

But modern childhood is not all bad: technology allows us to keep in touch and stay informed and entertained, and processed junk foods, like chicken nuggets, really can hit the spot when you've got hungry mouths to feed in a hurry.

As parents, although we want to help, with so much going on, opportunities for proper communication are reduced and this leaves many of us relying on snatched conversations on the way to school or just before bed, when enquiries about whether everything is okay might be met with little more than a grunt. It can be really difficult to find the right moment to connect and possibly step in with advice or support before a problem erupts into something bigger.

Great advances in the study of modern parenting over the last 30–40 years have shown that effective and sensitive parenting can have a deeply significant impact on your children's lives. The way we interact with our children really can make a huge difference to how confident, happy and healthy they are both now and long into their future. And one clever way to boost that positive interaction, while simultaneously establishing strong foundations of health, is finding time to cook and eat together as a family.

It can be all too easy to start thinking there's no point dicing a carrot or frying an onion when there are so many cheap and speedy alternatives that can be whipped out of the freezer and into the air fryer or the microwave in minutes. And that's a pity. It means those basic cooking skills and the confidence to throw a few things together to rustle up a home-cooked meal are becoming lost. Experts are also increasingly worried that our galloping over-reliance on ultra-processed foods (UPFs) is causing problems with our children's mental and physical health. Frighteningly, many children in the UK have a diet made up of around 60 per cent UPFs. These foods are typically high in calories, unhealthy fats, sugar, starch and salt, and are also made from food-like substances you wouldn't recognise in your kitchen. Eating UPFs means you could be consuming far too many artificial additives and preservatives, which have been shown to impact behaviour. Some studies have suggested a link between a diet high in UPFs and an increased risk of mental health issues, including depression and anxiety. A diet lacking in essential nutrients, and particularly protein and fibre, can affect a child's cognitive development and academic performance, with research showing that children whose diet is primarily composed of UPFs are also more likely to struggle with attention, memory and learning.

The addictive qualities of UPFs and the 'pester power' fostered by advertising targeted specifically at children mean that the more UPFs they eat, the more reluctant your children are likely to be to try, taste and enjoy the wide range of natural foods we need for good health.

Many Mediterranean countries, like Spain, still eat together as a family for at least two meals a week over 70 per cent of the time. Sadly, the UK has dropped to as low as 30 per cent of families managing to eat together twice a week. This omission is making the job of being a good parent so much harder. Preparing food and then cooking and eating together – even if you only manage to do it once a week– is such a fantastic opportunity to check in with your kids, to monitor their progress, and to watch out for early signs of any possible problems. It cuts back on their intake of harmful UPFs, too, and gives your children the chance to communicate with you and their siblings without the distraction of TV or phones. It also opens their eyes to the wonderful world of deliciously healthy real food.

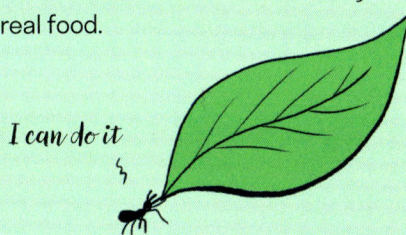

I can do it

The solution

Eating together is the key to happy families. We all want our children to live happy and fulfilled lives, to achieve their potential, enjoy a strong sense of identity, to share good family values and to go on to forge meaningful relationships in the future. And, as parents, we have considerable influence over the way our children turn out.

But when you're at the coal face, juggling work and family, possibly with financial pressures and plenty of stressors of your own, it can seem fiendishly difficult to know how to tread the right path.

However, decades of research have shown that effective parenting is so powerful it can dramatically transform your relationship with your child, improve their behaviour and set your children up for confidence and success in the future.

Yes, you might have been picking up a few tips watching TikTok, *Supernanny* on TV, or by following (or completely ignoring) advice from your own parents, but there is good scientific evidence to show the benefits of working to a simple formula that balances plenty of love (in the form of playing together, offering praise and listening to your child), with setting up and sticking to boundaries (the 'dos and don'ts' of good behaviour, which you explain clearly, and gently reinforce). For optimum health and development, children need a balance of both.

Working together, we have fine-tuned the balance of these two parenting parameters into a blueprint for effective parenting, which we call 'Love and Limits'. This concept is at the heart of the www.parentingmatters.co.uk online course we have pioneered, and it fundamentally reflects the beneficial practices outlined in this book.

Stephen's research with families and his many published studies provide scientific evidence that the combination of showing love and support to your child, while also establishing clear boundaries, is the best path to generating a close bond founded on mutual respect.

In an ideal world, we'd love every parent to take our course and start basing all their parenting decisions and actions on the principles of 'Love and Limits' but time, as we have identified, is VERY tight. However, if you can establish a habit of eating together as a family, you get a wealth of fantastic opportunities to pick up and practise these skills on a regular basis.

We hope this book will show you how to infuse your children's lives with an interest in healthy eating. It will hopefully encourage you all to gather around the table to eat meals together and, importantly, it will also show you how to polish your 'Love and Limits' parenting skills in the process, and help you transform your family dynamic now and into the future.

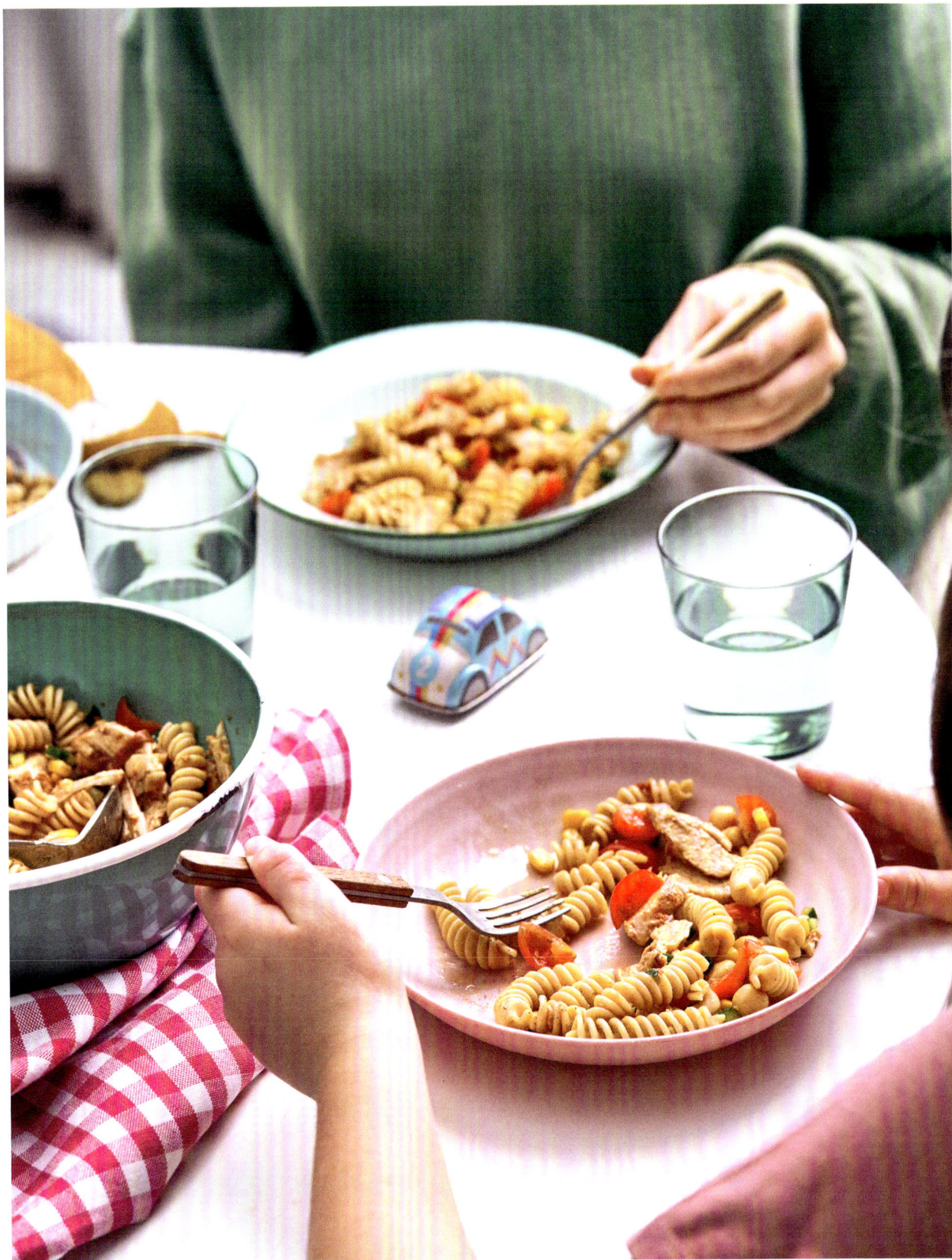

The right kind of love

We love our children. Of course we do. But it turns out the way we transmit that love can make a surprising difference to our children. We might show that love with gifts or treats, offering hugs or cuddles and telling them – as often as possible – just how much we love them. But, beyond that, research shows that the most powerful approach is 'sensitive responding'. This is a very subtle, yet very easy to implement, surprisingly effective part of the 'Love and Limits' parenting approach. Put simply, it means *responding sensitively* playing Minecraft with your friends' can get through to a teen gamer more powerfully than, 'You know we love you very much', but research shows that 'sensitive responding' seems to resonate deeply with young minds. It comforts children and helps them believe you really understand their emotions and what it's like to be them.

Another 'sensitive responding' technique is listening to your child and then repeating back to them what they've just said, but with added empathy for the emotions they might have expressed, or adding something from your

> Eating together, preparing food and cooking together with your children provide a wealth of wonderful opportunities to practise your 'sensitive responding' as a parenting skill.

to what your child is saying, thinking or doing. One great technique with young children is to 'act like a football commentator', where you offer a gentle, kind and positive commentary to whatever your child is doing, which is couched in mild praise. You might feel a little awkward hovering behind your child when they are playing with their toys, mumbling, 'Oh, you've connected the blue engine to the track, that's great to see how you're pushing the carriages along', or, 'I can see you've drawn a lovely face with a green nose', but, be under no doubt, this counts as good attention from you. It's about listening and following your child's lead and connecting at their level. It is the kind of 'love' children really need – and it has a deep impact.

Stephen's research shows that children of all ages love it! You might wonder how saying something like, 'You're having so much fun own experience. 'Oh, so you sat next to Zac at school today? What was that like?' And then, 'Zac was naughty? That must have made it hard for you to do your work?' And then, 'What shall we do about that? Do you think we should talk to your teacher about letting you sit somewhere else?' or, 'I remember the same thing happening to me when I was in year two.'

Practising this technique will strengthen your bond, which means your children will be more likely to tell you what's going on in their lives (good and bad). And because they trust you, they are more likely to listen to your advice.

For sensitive responding to work at its best, you should be fully focused on your child (facing towards them, giving them your full attention – no phones!). This is why it works so well when you are eating together; it gives you and your child that eye contact and vital warm connection.

Stephen's research shows that practising 'sensitive responding' for just 10 minutes a day is such a great way to engender a feeling of trust and closeness that children he studied go on to have better relationships, succeed at school and have greater self-confidence and resilience. It also shows that the knock-on effects can last a lifetime. In fact, there is a very powerful case for the widespread offering of early interventions that improve the quality of care-giving to children. These lead to better behavioural and health outcomes, and have even been shown to have a significant cost saving to society.

Furthermore, when sensitive responding for ten minutes a day is combined with setting clear, calm boundaries (see below), children settle down more easily to reading and homework, becoming more engaged in the task and concentrating better. This is proven by objective testing of reading skills and verbal intelligence after using the parenting strategies. In one study of six-year-olds, their reading age advanced by six months compared with those who did not use the strategies, and a similar strong effect was found in a second study. Moreover, these effects lasted into adolescence, so that teenagers whose parents had used the methods had a verbal IQ ten points higher than those who had not. So using this approach is a good investment for your children!

Eating together, preparing food and cooking together with your children provide a wealth of wonderful opportunities to practise your 'sensitive responding' as a parenting skill.

The importance of boundaries
It might sound a little contentious, but children – a bit like dogs and horses – are much happier when they know where the boundaries are. This doesn't mean you have to be a strict authoritarian, it's just a question of establishing clear 'limits' for various aspects of your life, which give you opportunities to lavish praise when they are met ('It was great that you held my hand when we were walking along that busy road!') and which can be backed up by consequences when needed.

We all have different parenting styles, which may vary according to the age and personality of our children. The approach we take is often determined by how we were brought up, our own personality, experiences, culture, or simply what we have picked up from those around us.

We have observed a growing trend for 'gentle parenting' with adults wanting to be 'friends' with their children. This can be confusing. The 12,000 parents who filled in the parenting style quiz on our www.parentingmatters.co.uk website have shown that as many as 60 per cent prefer an easy-going 'permissive' parenting style. But parents need to be able to have the authority to set boundaries and follow up consequences when needed. Being able to do that calmly and consistently is key. Children thrive within clear boundaries, and it makes life easer all round.

Studies (including a Demos Report called 'Building Character', which researched 9,000 families) show lifelong benefits of being brought up with what they call a 'well-balanced/authoritative' parenting style that combines warmth and encouragement along with clear consistent boundaries. These children were more likely to develop the qualities needed for modern life – including empathy, application and self-control. This means setting up a few rules (whether for your child's safety or just to make life easier for all of you) and being prepared to make sure they are adhered to.

If the idea of setting limits is new or difficult for you, this approach applies to eating together, too. Getting everyone together for cooking or preparing food, and ultimately eating together as a family, provides endless useful opportunities to set boundaries and to discuss consequences if those boundaries are breached. When it comes to eating together as a family, 'limits' might take the form of clear 'house rules' for helping out with the food preparation, getting involved with the cooking, various tasks in setting the table and clearing away, and the kind of behaviour you expect or hope for during a family meal ('no phones at the table' or 'no one gets down from the table without asking'). And, of course, lavishing praise when those limits are met.

The best way to introduce the idea of limits is to call a mini family meeting with both parents and say something like, 'Mum/Dad is doing all the work in the kitchen to get dinner ready each night, wouldn't it be great if we all give her/him a bit of a hand?' You can then chat about how the various tasks could be divided up (even the youngest children can get involved, perhaps just by stirring a wooden spoon in a saucepan). It might help to set up a star chart that offers 'rewards' for each time help is offered. Or you could say that any refusal to help will result in a 10-minute cut in screen time.

It is easier to enforce boundaries when the rules are pre-set so everyone knows what is expected. It's a good idea to stick a chart on the fridge laying things out. You need to lead by example! For instance, it is perfectly reasonable to get the children involved in laying the table, clearing away or helping to stack the dishwasher afterwards, but with smaller children aim to give very clear and specific instructions. Rather than say, 'Please lay the table', it helps to break the task down into small, specific steps: 'Please go to the drawer and take out three forks, three knives and three spoons.' If they don't comply within a few seconds, Stephen suggests putting your hand on their shoulder and leading them to the drawer. And then, as soon as they've done each task, be quick to offer praise ('Thank you for getting the cutlery ready for the table').

It can help to think through possible 'consequences' that can be calmly applied if the limits are rebuffed (perhaps a quarter or half hour reduction in TV time?). To get them going, you might consider a reward chart as incentive (one star for every time they help, or for sitting at the table for 20 minutes, which adds up to a treat at the end of the week). So, you might say, 'Hey! Let's get dinner ready!' And then follow this up with, 'Ruben, could you help me peel the potatoes?' If you get a negative response, you can be firmer: 'I'd like you to help me peel the potatoes, please.' And gently guide them towards the kitchen with, 'Come on, it will be fun and it'll only take five minutes.'

Consequences should not be too draconian. ('If you don't turn the TV off when I ask, tomorrow night's TV time will be reduced by half,' rather than, 'Right! We're getting rid of the TV!') They should be gentle but impactful.

Aim to give a gentle warning that a 'limit' is being (or about to be) breached, and then give lashings of praise whenever your child complies with the new regime. ('Well done for turning off your game and joining us.' Or, 'I noticed you stopped as soon as I asked.')

To really make the 'limits' stick, any consequences should be consistently and swiftly applied (within the next 24 hours). It may take some determination on your part to see the consequences through (children will inevitably test you, especially if they have become used to getting their own way).

By remaining calm as you give instructions, and applying gentle consequences if they are not followed through, you will be providing your child with invaluable skills they'll need for fitting in with other people and thriving at school.

And, as a parent, don't think you are above the 'Love and Limits' law. Everyone in the family should stick to the rules!

A chance to eat well
When you encourage children to eat together as a family – even if you aren't particularly focusing on healthy eating – the studies show their diet improves. Frequent family meals are associated with higher intakes of fruit and vegetables, and lower intakes of fast food and takeaway food, regardless of socioeconomic circumstances. Children who grow up having family dinners tend to eat more healthily and have lower rates of obesity in adulthood. Beyond that, children in families who eat together have better vocabularies, do better at school, are likely to have less anxiety and, as adults, have fewer mental health issues. Eating together is a powerful recipe!

We all know we should be limiting our consumption of ultra-processed foods and this is much more likely to happen if we are eating a homemade shepherd's pie (ideally with hidden vegetables blended in with the mince – see page 129), or a chicken stir fry with noodles (see page 132) just once or twice a week. With rising concerns about childhood obesity, it is reassuring to note that studies show eating together helps make weight control easier, too. Researchers in Canada found family meals also had such a powerful effect on children's wellbeing, they recommended the concept as a way to 'optimise child development'. The mental health benefits of eating together are very impressive. According to Dr Anne Fishel, who is professor of psychology at Harvard Medical School (and author of *The Family Dinner Project*), 'Regular family dinners are associated with lower rates of depression, and anxiety, and substance abuse. What's more, it is also found to be linked to fewer eating disorders, less tobacco use, reduced early teenage pregnancy, along with higher rates of resilience and better self-esteem.'

A survey in 2022 by the American Heart Association found 91 per cent of parents said their family is less stressed when they eat together. The vast majority (84 per cent) of respondents said they wish they could share a meal more often with loved ones, and nearly all parents surveyed reported lower levels of stress among their family when they were able to connect regularly over a meal.

Eating together is just one thing, yet it can have a powerful and far-reaching effect.

The best advice is to eat together as often as you can and to do what you can to make those mealtimes fun and engaging. Cook from scratch if and when you can – it is cheaper, more nutritious and it tastes better. The recipes in the second part of this book will leave you spoiled for choice.

WHAT TO FEED THE KIDS

- **When planning meals**, prioritise protein (meat, fish, eggs, pulses) and fibre (vegetables, salad, fruit). Protein is needed for the healthy function of your biological systems and it makes meals more filling. As a guide, a child should aim to eat protein at every meal, whether that's grated cheese, chicken, yoghurt or eggs. Aim for a portion roughly the size of their palm. Turn to page 203 for some ideas on how to top up your child's protein – and your own!

- **Variety** is the key to getting a good balance of nutrients in your diet, so aim to eat a rainbow of differently coloured fruits and vegetables to get a really wide spread of the anti-inflammatory phytonutrients.

- **Where you can**, try to add greens to each meal and include brown rice, quinoa, bulgur wheat or beans and pulses to add fibre and important nutrients.

- **Switch** from highly processed 'white' carbohydrates (rice, pasta, noodles, bread) to wholegrain or brown alternatives that contain beneficial fibre and nutrients. These will keep your children fuller for longer.

- **Increase** your fibre intake gradually to avoid uncomfortable bloating, which can happen if your gut microbes aren't used to processing fibre. Once you have switched from white bread and pasta to brown varieties, start to add a few beans to your stew and lentils, seeds or nuts to a salad.

- **Gradually reduce** your children's consumption of sugar and sugary foods. Their taste buds will adapt (and you'll find plenty of sugar-free and low-sugar treats in this book).

- **Gradually dilute** sweet drinks until your children are happy drinking water. Plain water always tastes better when chilled or flavoured with a slice of fresh lemon, a few mint leaves or berries. Offer whole milk instead of high-calorie drinks.

- **Dramatically reduce** the number of ultra-processed foods and sweetened drinks you offer your kids.

- **Aim to serve** one meal for everyone; don't offer alternatives without a good reason.

- **Avoid** becoming a self-service food provider – it can be so easy to feed each child food you know they will eat, but this limits their exposure to new foods and creates a lot of hard work for you. Instead, offer limited choices: 'This one or that?'

IMPORTANT NUTRIENTS FOR GROWING CHILDREN

- **OMEGA-3:** This is particularly important for your child's brain development and is mostly found in oily fish, such as salmon, mackerel and sardines, as well as in chia seeds, flaxseed and walnuts, seaweed and algae.

- **IRON:** An essential mineral for red blood cell formation, energy and preventing anaemia, but it is also needed for brain development. Good sources include lean meats, beans, fortified cereals and leafy greens.

- **VITAMIN D:** Key for bone health and immune function, vitamin D is absorbed naturally through the skin in sunlight and is also found in fortified dairy products, fatty fish and egg yolks.

- **CALCIUM:** Vital for the development of bones and teeth, calcium also supports muscle function. Dairy products, leafy greens and fortified plant-based milks are sources.

- **VITAMIN A:** Great for eye health, skin and immunity, vitamin A is found in orange vegetables and green leafy vegetables.

- **MAGNESIUM:** Useful for energy, muscle and bone health, this mineral is found in nuts, seeds, whole grains and leafy greens.

- **ZINC:** Necessary for growth, immunity and healing, zinc is sourced in meats, beans and whole grains.

Shopping and planning

When we think about the wonderful positive parenting opportunities presented by eating together as a family, we probably imagine the happy scenes of our childhood with everyone sitting around a table tucking into a delicious home-cooked meal. That's certainly a fantastic aspirational goal.

But luckily, it turns out there is MUCH to be offered and gained from every small step you take to get there. Just by encouraging children to be a little more involved in the whole eating process – whether that's a little bit of meal planning, food shopping or cooking together – you can boost their exposure to new skills and healthy eating, and you get so many wonderful opportunities to practise effective parenting skills to help you bond as a family and set up your children for life. For a start, there are numerous health benefits to be had from helping children get a better

not just breaded nuggets!), and the huge variety of options available (red and green, small and large, tart and sweet apples). Not to mention teaching them about costs and perhaps digging into the whole concept of seasonality, along with the pros and cons of buying locally sourced produce.

When you involve your children with meal planning, you are including them in the family team and, even if they might groan about being dragged away from the TV, this involvement can make them feel grown up and important.

By encouraging children to be involved in the eating process – whether that's meal planning, food shopping or cooking together – you can boost their exposure to new skills and healthy eating.

understanding of food and trying to make the concept of healthy eating fun.

For instance, by chatting with children about food and getting them involved in the shopping and meal prep, you will be imparting important information about where food really comes from (milk from a cow not a carton!), what it looks like in its various forms (whole chicken, chicken breasts, thighs and mince –

Shopping and planning meals together is also a chance to outline safe 'limits' and to offer rewards when children comply, as well as constructive consequences when they don't. If your child is running around the supermarket, you might ask them to stay nearby or put one hand on the trolley (this is their 'boundary'). Praise them when they comply. This process is always much more helpful if you can give very clear instructions followed by loads of encouragement and praise. Try to keep everything FUN and children will very quickly learn that compliance can be enjoyable and rewarding.

Getting the children involved is also a great way to encourage your child's curiosity about different foods. It's good to let them 'play' with the food as you prepare a meal together, feeling the different textures, smells, shapes and colours, and offer tiny pieces to be sniffed, licked and tasted. You can turn the volume up on the fun element by joining in the tasting, too, offering your thoughts, like a sommelier picking up hints and flavours in fine wine.

If you're pushed for time, it can be tempting to shoo young children out from under your feet, but studies show that getting the children involved in the meal preparation not only makes the most of the limited time everyone has, but it also appears to strengthen the many benefits that shared meals offer. The key is giving clear, calm instructions and being lavish with the praise and appreciation. And for younger children, put a positive gloss on their actions as you describe them out loud, to boost their confidence and connection, and to make them feel good about what you are doing together. (See more about this on page 14.)

Give each child individual responsibilities depending on their age and abilities, no matter how young they are. They will learn useful skills and (eventually) become helpful and competent. The added bonus? With an army of helpers, you are less likely to feel like the family dogsbody when it comes to putting food on the table!

FIVE WAYS TO GET THE KIDS INVOLVED

1 Lunchbox pick 'n' mix
If your children take a packed lunch to school, encourage them to take a bit of shared ownership of what goes into it each day. You could start with a chat about the importance of protein and fibre (see page 18) to help keep them feeling full, and discuss the problems with too much sugar whizzing them up and creating energy crashes. This might be an opportunity to suggest a fun session cooking healthy cakes or biscuits together at the weekend (see recipes on pages 180–99), so you can wrap and freeze individual slices ready for grabbing as a healthy on-the-go snack or to pop into their lunchbox. This way, children can learn to compile their own nutritionally balanced lunchbox combos that contain protein, such as meat, cheese, eggs, fish or pulses, as well as fibre, in the form of whole grains, vegetable sticks, salad or fruit.

2 Recipe pot luck
Get together with older children to plan meals for the upcoming week. Each member of the family could pick a meal they enjoy (or a recipe from this book) to be eaten on a day when they have a little time to help prepare and cook. This process gives children some agency over what they're eating. If you can only manage one meal together each week, let them take it in turns to choose the meal and take some responsibility for encouraging the others to enjoy it. It's all about getting them interested in trying new things.

3 Supermarket treasure hunt

When it comes to food shopping, put away all nightmarish thoughts of dragging the children around the supermarket when everyone is hungry and tired, and all the cupboards at home are bare. That's too stressful for all of you!

I remember as a child we were deployed as 'fetchers' by my mother, who would whisk the supermarket trolley up and down the aisles instructing us to go and find whatever food item she requested. We would then throw it into the fast-moving trolley. It was like playing basketball and great fun!

In fact, my mother, who was herself a child psychiatrist, was cleverly keeping us occupied and giving us a sense of responsibility. We treated it a bit like a treasure hunt, and my mother had a willing band of helpers to speed up the shopping process.

Possibly more rewarding, and more in keeping with the 'Love and Limits' philosophy, would be to make a special shopping trip, perhaps with just one of your children if you have a large brood. Keep it short and aim to find lots of opportunities to notice praiseworthy behaviour.

If they're old enough, the child could practise writing out the shopping list – explaining what each item is – and you could go to the shop together. You could send them off to find items from the shopping list, or try setting up a game of 'find me a red apple/ wonky carrot' or 'bring me a piece of fruit you've never seen before', and then put a few unfamiliar new foods into your basket so you can try them later at home.

When you get home from shopping, talk about the foods' texture, smell, colour and taste. This is particularly beneficial for fussy eaters – the more often they get to touch, feel and smell different foods, the more familiar they become and the more likely they will be to embrace them when they land on their plate.

4 Going solo

As children get older, it's good to give them a sense of responsibility for food shopping. Start by hanging back and asking them to take a basket of food through the checkout when you are shopping together. This is a great opportunity for a positive commentary and lots of encouragement.

On another occasion, you could wait outside the shop and send them in to find and buy one or two items on their own – then shower them with praise for their achievement afterwards. You will be demonstrating that you trust your child, and will be making them feel capable and grown up. This is a great way to help develop their resilience.

5 Online shoptastic

It is worthwhile getting your children involved with the online shop, too. Perhaps you can ask them to scroll through the options and pick one fruit and one vegetable they've never tried before. You can try their chosen items together, experimenting with different ways to prepare and taste them. Or show them how much more expensive one type of tomato is than another type, and suggest you buy both as an experiment – a blindfolded taste test to see if anyone can taste the difference.

When the food delivery arrives, ask the children to help you put things away (it's a great opportunity to teach them about why some foods need refrigerating).

STORE CUPBOARD BASICS

Stock your kitchen cupboards and freezer with healthy staples and you will always have easy, nutritious options at hand to throw together for a last-minute meal.

- **CANS:** Chopped tomatoes, cooked white and black beans, cooked chickpeas, sweetcorn, fish (such as salmon, sardines and tuna), fruit in juice rather than syrup (such as pears, peaches and apricots) and coconut cream.

- **JARS:** Anchovies, peanut butter, coconut oil, red peppers (capsicums), passata, mayonnaise, gherkins, Dijon mustard, sun-dried tomato pesto, tomato paste, honey, maple syrup and vanilla extract.

- **NUTS:** Walnuts, cashews, pistachios, desiccated coconut, flaked almonds and blanched hazelnuts.

- **DRIED FOODS:** Rolled oats, ground almonds, spelt flour, wholegrain flour, red lentils, wholegrain pasta and rice, baking powder, cocoa powder, dark chocolate (with over 70% cocoa solids), pitted dates and sultanas.

- **SPICES:** Chilli flakes, cinnamon, ground nutmeg, paprika, curry powder, stock cubes, mixed spice and mixed herbs.

- **SEEDS:** Chia seeds, flaxseed, sesame seeds and mixed seeds.

- **FROZEN FOODS:** Prawns, peas, spinach and berries.

- **SAUCES:** Olive oil, soy sauce, balsamic vinegar, Worcestershire sauce and sriracha.

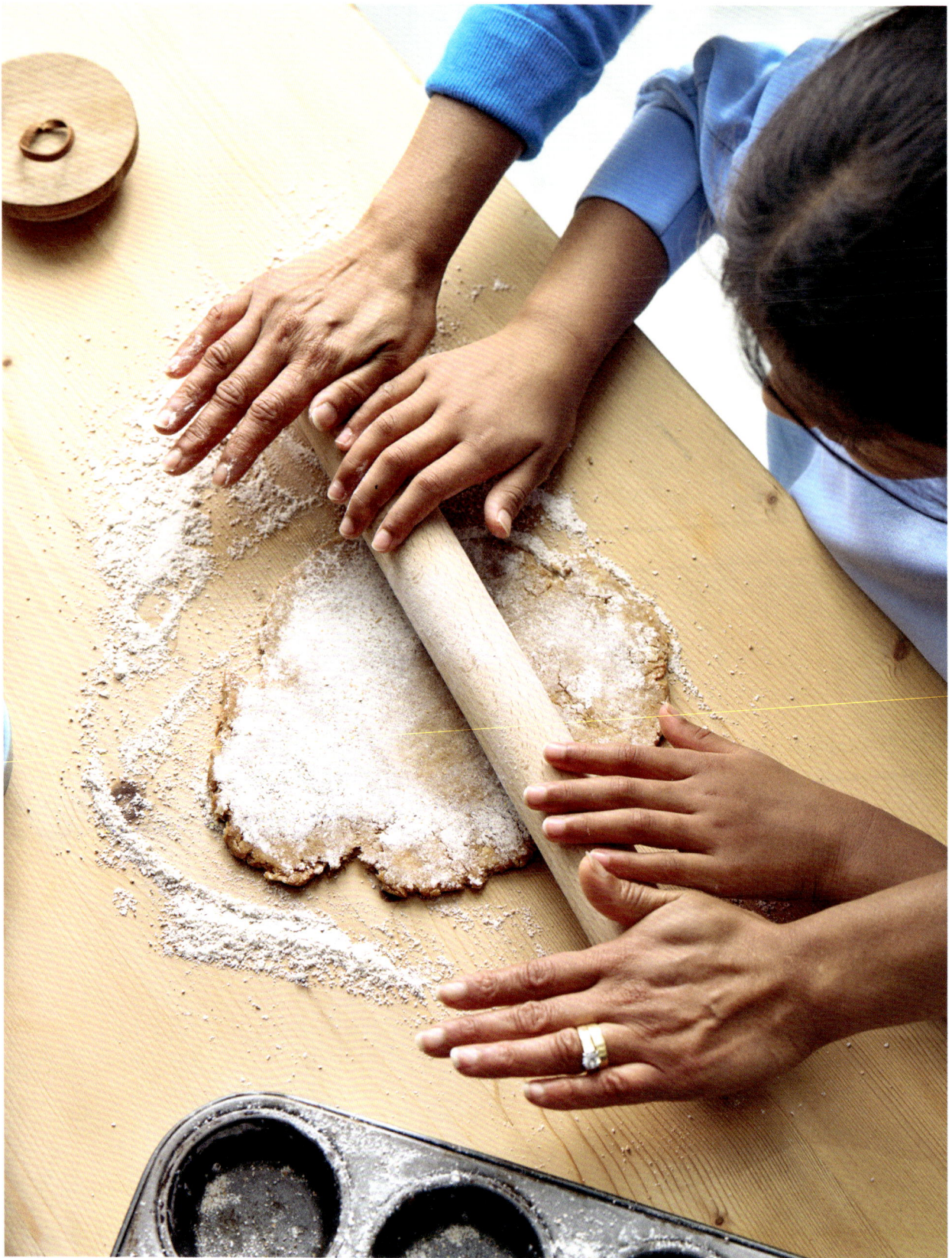

Cooking together

If the thought of getting the whole family around the table to eat the same meal still feels like a 'someday, maybe' fairytale, then you can be quietly confident that by spending just a few minutes cooking with the children you will have taken the first step in the right direction.

Cooking together – whether that's boiling an egg, rolling out biscuit dough or fine-tuning the flavour profile of a slow-cooked stew – is a truly fantastic opportunity to expand a child's food horizons. It exposes them to new nutrients and flavours, builds the confidence they might need to feed themselves independently, encourages them to follow instructions (recipes) and collaborate (with you and their siblings).

How many people do you know who say they can't or won't cook because they just don't to be part of the family team – to contribute and learn new skills. Cooking together also provides plenty of opportunities for you to practise the principles of 'Love and Limits' and so intensify your growing bond.

No matter how busy you are, you should be able to find time for one of the really quick, definite hits in this book, such as Instant Apple and Chocolate Pudding (see page 189), which takes only three minutes to prepare and less than two minutes to cook in the microwave. It's a chance to share the joy of creating

> Cooking together provides plenty of opportunities for you to practise the principles of 'Love and Limits' and so intensify your growing bond.

know how? That often happens if they weren't exposed to a bit of cooking at home as a child.

But even if you don't know a spatula from a colander, it's never too late to start! If you're not the most confident cook yourself, the thought of having the children 'helping' you in the kitchen might sound rather messy and a recipe for chaos, but young children really are hard-wired to be helpful – or at least what they see as helpful. They desperately want something together and to focus on a shared goal. It is also a lovely opportunity to look out for a chance to praise your child – perhaps for finding all the ingredients, or for passing you the tea towel. Any gentle challenge, no matter how small, unobtrusively allows youngsters to hone their problem-solving skills. The more you include the children, the more competent they will become, and you will soon find that you can enlist them to help properly.

Whenever you are in the kitchen, encourage the kids to join in as part of the family food-production team – chopping vegetables, stirring a pot, lining a baking tray – depending on their age and ability. Let them roll their sleeves up and get their hands messy. You might be surprised at how willingly they join you, especially when you find opportunities to lavish praise on them.

A food-loving friend remembers hating white sauce and rejecting any food with a sauce until her mother showed her how to make one – stirring the butter, flour and milk, and watching it transform. It altered her taste expectations, as well as introducing a valuable new culinary skill.

children important life skills. Once they've mastered Shepherd's Pie (see page 129) and Sneaky Spag Bol (see page 125), both packed with hidden vegetables, they'll be set up for living on their own. And, by the time they fly the nest, the veg won't have to be hidden!

Start them young

Younger children can help – even if it is just stirring a wooden spoon around in an empty pan. Put an apron on any child and they instantly think they're the chef! If you guide them properly and offer supervision, children can stand at the hob stirring a sauce, jointly hold a blitzer or even chop vegetables (you can buy kitchen safety knives quite cheaply

> Younger children can help – even if it is just stirring a wooden spoon around in an empty pan. Put an apron on any child and they instantly think they're the chef!

If you've got a vegetable refuser in your brood, you might find that helping to prepare one element of an evening meal builds intrigue that helps to overcome the fear of trying something new. That's why I've included a selection of clever recipes (Garlicky Green Beans on page 157, Roasted Pesto and Parmesan Pumpkin on page 144, and even Baked Spinach with Parmesan on page 150), which transform humble vegetables to make them more tantalising.

Not only is cooking together a lovely inclusive exercise that helps you bond and gives opportunities to chat about anything and everything, you can bask in the slightly smug glow of knowing you are teaching your

to allow young children to join in with the food preparation without risk of cutting themselves). If your children love cheese, a rotary grater allows them to grate cheese without touching the grating blades. Kids love stirring, drizzling oil, buttering, decorating and spooning. Get them creating fillings for wraps, and all children are fascinated by the chance to crack eggs.

Try to allow lots of time to chat, with plenty of opportunities to listen and ask questions as you work together.

Breakfast like a king

A good starting point for kitchen newbies might be to get everyone together to prepare healthy breakfast options on a lazy weekend morning when there's a lot less pressure on your time. The sweetened breakfast cereal companies have had everything their own way for far too long and those highly processed nuggets are contributing to our children's potentially toxic UPF load. Your children are much more likely to accept a healthy breakfast alternative if they've played a part in preparing and cooking it themselves – try the delicious Strawberry Chia Pots on page 58. These creamy pots will keep children full for longer, thanks to protein in the Greek yoghurt and fibre in the chia seeds. And your kids are more likely to think about switching cereal for overnight oats (see page 53) if they've had a fun evening

183) and Apricot Traybake (see page 187) – have a low-sugar, healthy twist.

Training young masterchefs
Older children will find many of the recipes in this book can be made with minimal supervision (just a little loving attention) and will enjoy the autonomy of producing something on their own. Ask teenagers to flick through the recipes and find a meal they'd like to cook – this gives them an element of choice and control, and they'll have a great sense of pride in their achievement. You could perhaps be adventurous and suggest each teenager take responsibility for food on a different night when they don't have any after-school clubs to go to.

> Older children will find many of the recipes in this book can be made with minimal supervision and will enjoy the autonomy of producing something on their own.

in the kitchen the night before putting the ingredients together. There's so much to be gained from working collaboratively to make pancakes (see page 63), porridge (see page 57) or cheesy eggy bread (see page 67), and everyone will be getting wholesome nutrients that will keep them feeling full all the way up until lunchtime.

Family bake off
What child doesn't enjoy making cakes with their mum or dad? Sweet treats are a great way to tempt reluctant cooks into the kitchen, and all of the treat recipes in this book – such as Oaty Chocolate Cookies (see page 180), Sweet Potato Hot Cross Brownies (see page

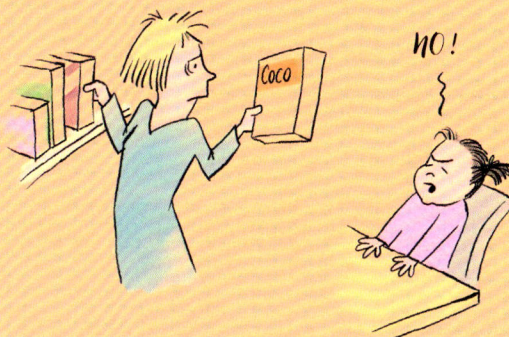

Eating together

The idea of eating together means different things to different families. It might be a completely new and scary concept for you. If you rarely ate together as a family when you were a child, it can be difficult to imagine how you're going to get the rest of the family to agree to the idea.

It is so easy to fall into the habit of eating in front of the TV, and the thought of persuading the children – or even your partner – to sit down at the same time, eat the same food and interact with each other can seem impossible.

But I cannot emphasise enough how important and how beneficial eating together can be for your children's mental and physical health, as well as for establishing a strong connection between you all as a family unit.

Although it might seem challenging when you're not used to doing it, think of each meal

Lay the foundations of getting the family to eat together, by starting to involve the children in food shopping and preparation (see pages 20–2). Better still, get them to help you out with a bit of cooking, too (see pages 25–7). The ideal situation would be to get everyone so excited that they can't wait for the chance to share the food they've been helping to prepare.

It's also a good idea to clear away as many potential barriers as possible before you start. So, if you've got a dining table buried in 'stuff', try to clear the space so it's more welcoming.

Think of each meal together as quality, ring-fenced family time that offers a respite from the hustle-bustle of everyday life.

together as quality, ring-fenced family time that offers a respite from the hustle-bustle of everyday life. It is a wonderful opportunity to create an environment where you enjoy food together, conversations are meaningful and fun, and you can prioritise healthy food choices. It is a key time for bonding – your children will learn that you are there for them, you can pick up on any worries they may have, and you can have space to chat, connect and build relationships.

Make sure you've got enough chairs at the correct heights so everyone can reach (use cushions or a highchair for younger ones). And if you don't have table space, think about how you might have a picnic on the floor, or arrange the living room so you can all sit facing each other (rather than facing the TV).

Turn the page to find out how to create the regular habit of a harmonious family meal from scratch in just four weeks by taking things one step at a time.

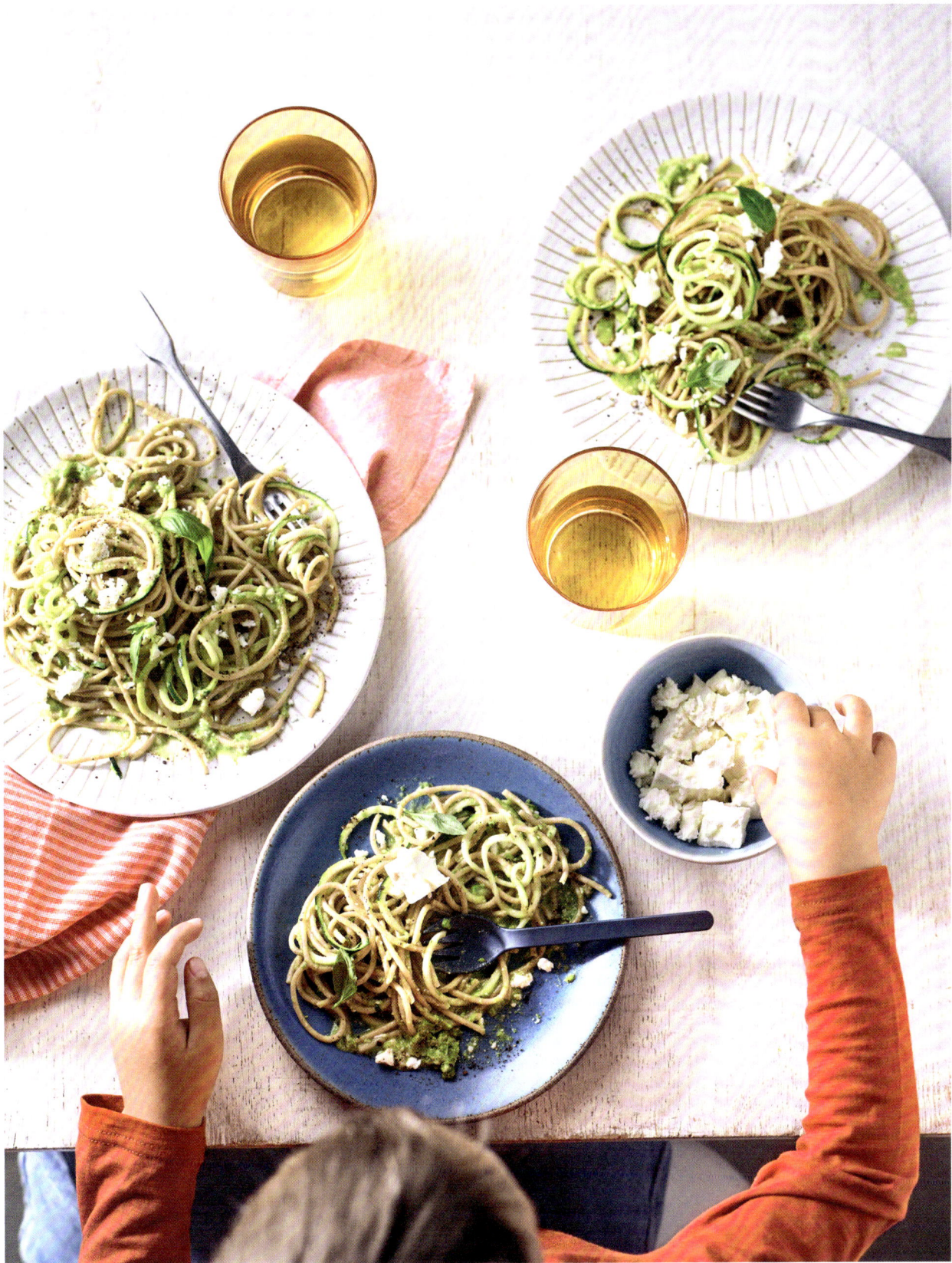

The four-week plan

WEEK ONE | Sow the seeds of the idea

1 First, set the scene. Call a five-minute family meeting at a time when everyone is under the same roof and say you'd really like to start planning a family meal because you'd love everyone to eat together and tell stories about their day. Keep the whole conversation light and positive. This family meal has to sound like it's going to be loads of FUN and a bit special.

2 If this is a completely alien concept to your children and you suspect you might meet some resistance, it could help to kick things off by pinpointing a day when you have something to celebrate: 'It's my birthday next week and this is the best present I could wish for.' 'Granny is coming to stay at the weekend – wouldn't it be wonderful to make her feel special?'

3 Agree on a day and time and encourage everyone to get involved with the planning so the children feel an element of control, and no one is left out: 'How do you think we should do this?' 'What would you like to eat?' 'Which day would work best?' 'What time shall we do this so you don't miss your favourite TV show?' 'What can we do to really make this fun?'

4 Talking about the family meal first and setting the scene makes it far more likely to be successful than if it were announced out of the blue, forcing the children to tear themselves away from the comfort and familiarity of eating in front of the TV.

5 When it comes to planning what you're going to eat, there's absolutely no need to worry about making it super healthy at this stage. It will probably be easier if you stick to firm favourites, such as Parmesan-crusted Fish Nuggets (see page 120). Try to encourage everyone to agree on ONE meal choice that both the adults and children can tuck into. If someone complains that it isn't their favourite dish at that first meal, reassure them that they won't be expected to eat the whole lot, but suggest their favourite is chosen for the next family meal.

6 Delegate responsibilities so everyone feels involved: 'Jake, would you like to pick a recipe from this book?' 'Sarah, would you like to come shopping with me to get the bits we need?' 'Tom, as you're so good at colouring, would you make invitations and place settings for everyone?' Shower praise on every tiny glimmer of enthusiasm (ignore any dissent). Make sure that everyone has a role and is actively participating.

7 You might meet a little resistance, but stick to your guns, be firm and say this family meal matters a lot to you and that it is a first-time experiment. The aim is to create a buzz of excitement about eating together so everyone in the family is talking about it.

WEEK TWO | The first family meal

1 For this first family meal, aim to keep everything really simple. No complex menu, nothing too fancy that might spark dissent. It doesn't matter if you're all eating pizza. The aim is to create a positive, fun event that the children enjoy and feel interested to repeat.

2 Keep the meal short, say 15–20 minutes, and try to ensure that everyone has a chance to speak. Aim to get everyone chatting about their favourite bits of eating together. What are they enjoying most? What do they like about the food? And if there were one thing each of them could change about the meal, what would it be? Ask the children about their day, one by one, and focus on really listening, to show that you are truly engaged with what they are saying.

3 Begin to sow the seeds of getting together for another family meal next week, and try to generate as much enthusiasm as you can muster for the idea: 'What day do you think works best?' 'What shall we eat?' 'Shall we make puddings together for the next meal?' 'Wouldn't that be fabulous?'

4 The key to ongoing success at this early stage is dishing out praise to everyone and anyone. This means being really attentive and looking out for tiny signs that a child is being helpful or kind to their siblings. You get extra parenting points for using the words 'I noticed' a lot: 'I noticed you're being really happy about this family meal idea.' 'I noticed you've been sitting really nicely.'

5 Finish by saying how much you've enjoyed eating together, how happy it has made you and list as many other good things as you can spot.

WEEK THREE | The second family meal

1 Call another family meeting to discuss the next get-together a few days after the first. Encourage the children to get involved with deciding which day and time works best, and gather ideas for what the children might like to eat. This second meal is less likely to be a big celebration, but it still needs to be fun, and the kids might want to continue some of the routines and traditions started at the first meal. The more positive and encouraging you are, the more successful you are likely to be at getting everyone on board.

2 This time you could ask for help with planning and preparation, teach the kids how to lay the table and give each their own task to be praised for, in order to generate more enthusiasm: 'I'm so glad you're as excited as I am about this!' 'It makes me so happy that you're helping me plan our family meal.'

3 Once you've built the strong foundations of positivity and everyone is on message and enjoying the idea of eating together, it's time to introduce a few gentle boundaries. Children of all ages need the structure of rules and consistent boundaries, even if they don't much like them, as they make them feel secure.

4 It is a good idea to chat about and agree on a few 'house rules' and explain why each rule is practical (specifically how it benefits the children as well as the adults around the table), and establish gentle but meaningful consequences that will be applied if the rules are not met. For example, you can make it a minimum requirement that everyone has a job to do, whether that's a bit of food prep, stirring a sauce, bringing the plates to the table, collecting up the cutlery at the end of the meal or putting a bowl in the sink. Other boundaries might include: everyone is expected to stay at the table until the end of the meal; everyone gets the chance to speak; no TV or phones at the table; everyone is to be nice to each other.

5 You might want to get one of the older children to write down the *Eating Together* Rules so they can be stuck on the fridge. Make a game of the fact that the rules apply to EVERYONE, even Mum and Granny!

6 Keep up with the fulsome praise: 'You held your knife and fork so well!' 'It was brilliant that you put a few peas in your mouth!' 'Thank you so much for asking me about my day.' Your new boundaries will also provide lots of opportunities for praise: 'You're being so kind to your brother!' 'Thank you for asking your Dad about his day.'

7 Try to stay calm and positive at the meal table. Ignore silly, irritating behaviours. Be patient, and remember that your children (and possibly your partner) are still learning!

8 Before the end of the meal, turn the conversation to how much you enjoyed the experience, asking everyone to name their favourite parts of the meal and to make suggestions for anything they might like to change next time.

WEEK FOUR | Making eating together a regular event

1 With luck – and quite a bit of effort on your part – eating together will have become a positive experience, and you should feel ready to start making it a regular event. The final task, therefore, is to make eating together a routine fixture – once, twice or even more times each week. Routines provide a reassuring structure that children love, and each family meal is an opportunity for you to interact and bond. So, the more family meals you can fit into your week, the better!

2 Pick a day and time that works for everyone. An evening meal together would be wonderful, but weekdays might be impossible if both parents work, so try to ring-fence a one-off midday or evening slot at the weekend, which could grow to become a regular fixture.

3 At every meal together, gradually build up the time spent at the table and slowly introduce new foods and more adventurous recipes. It's a good idea to keep checking in with the family, asking about the pros and cons of each meal together, taking any suggestions – even from the youngest children – seriously.

4 Sometimes eating together will be a quick weekend breakfast or a 30-minute kitchen dinner during the week, when you all come together before going off in different directions. But the more you show love and shower praise, the more the children will enjoy these family meals and start to really look forward to them.

5 Aim to reschedule any movable events or commitments to make it easier for these family meals to happen. Ideally, stick to a regular time for the meal. Aiming to eat meals at roughly the same time each day helps to create a predictable rhythm that can be reassuring for children and makes life easier over time.

Congratulations! After following this four-week plan you should be able to have one, or ideally more, regular family meals each week.

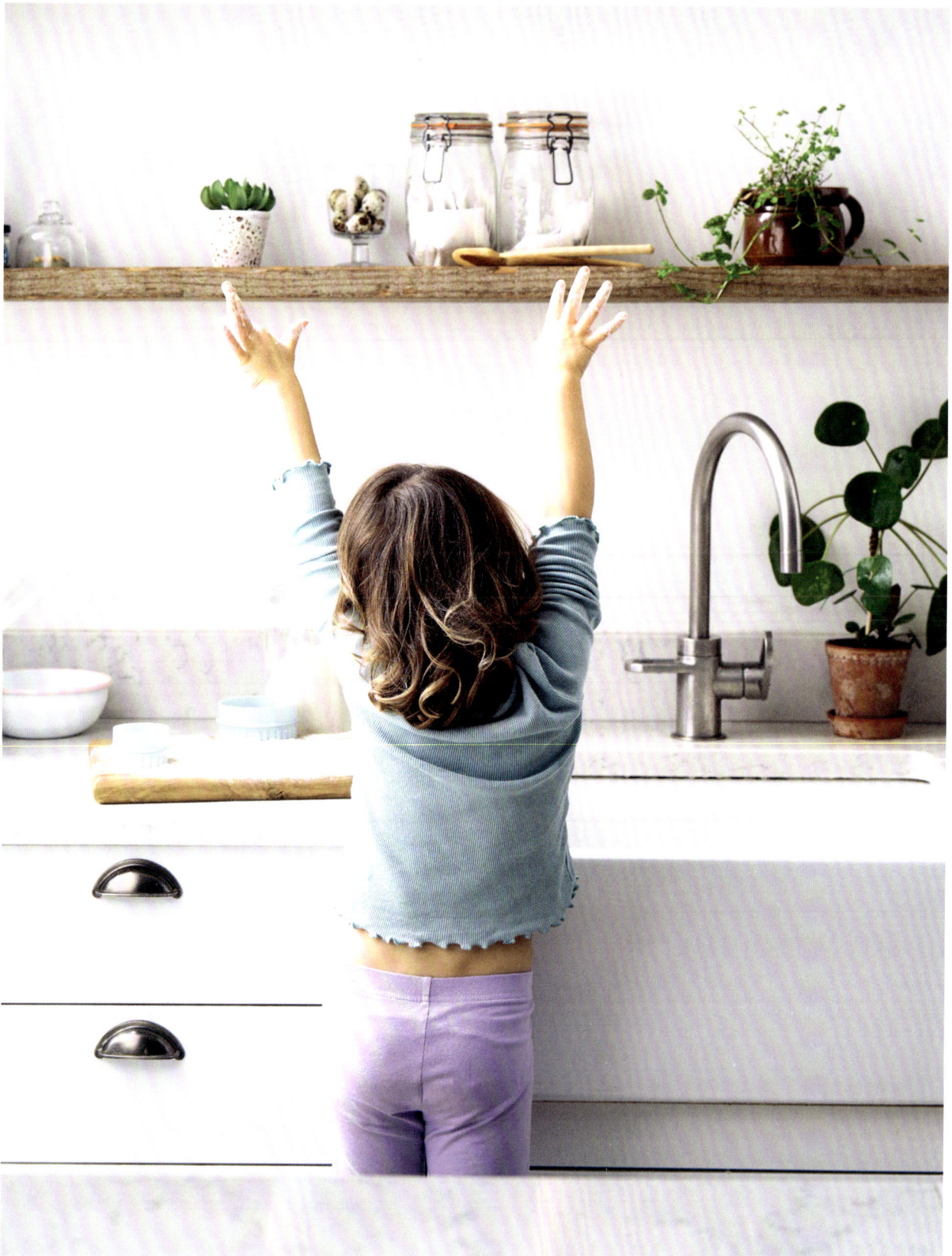

Kids just want to have fun!

The key to getting everyone back around the table, time after time, lies in making it fun. Try to create a positive environment – chat, play simple word games and get the conversation going. Aim to keep the atmosphere light and try to avoid arguments or confrontation – schedule those for a later time. Playing silly games (see pages 38–9) can help with bonding and can also distract a fussy eater and move the focus away from potential food battles.

Keep your expectations low. It takes time to change habits and you'll need to be realistic about the amount of time you expect a child to sit still – keep their age in mind. Do what you can to ensure your child is comfortable and included and, as they get used to the idea of eating together and become more and more engaged with the process, you'll find they will be happy to sit for longer.

If you have a very slow eater, it can derail the fun experience for everyone else. Don't expect them to finish what they are eating and quietly remove the plate after 20–30 minutes. You can always put a cover over it and let them know the food will be there if they feel hungry later.

It is crucial that you set a good example as children will take their lead from the adults around them. If you celebrate different foods, don't use mobile phones while you eat and do everything to make mealtimes calm and nurturing, they are likely to do so, too. Eighty per cent of your child's learning is from looking at what you do – so they will absorb your habits!

Sharing the love

Eating together on a regular basis – even if that's just a weekend breakfast or a Sunday lunch – will become family time that provides many wonderful opportunities for you all to interact and bond. You can really make the most of this regular opportunity to hone your parenting skills. The key lies in making meals a time when you talk together: tell the children what you've been doing and listen to what happened in their day. You'll get a better response and a more meaningful conversation if you ask detailed questions. Instead of asking, 'What did you do at school today?' try to be more specific: 'Who did you play with at break today?' 'How is your science project working out?' If you have more than one child, try to address each one in turn and encourage them to chip in with their own reactions to the person who is speaking (praise them when they do). Show great interest and be positive and sympathetic. Say 'Thank you' when they tell you what their day has been like.

You can get extra parenting points if you use the opportunity presented by family mealtimes to talk about feelings: 'How did you feel when . . .' 'That must have been horrible scary/annoying/upsetting.' And show a genuine interest. This will encourage your children to speak about what's on their mind and what's going on in their lives. Studies show that talking about and sharing emotions helps build self-esteem in children. By listening to what they have to say, it shows you value and respect what they think and do.

Take every chance to praise your child for sitting nicely, or for using a knife and fork, for being helpful to a younger sibling, and for trying new foods. If you aren't already doing it, give them appropriate tasks to help prepare food or set the table as part of the 'team'. Shower them with praise for tasks completed or for helping prepare, serve and clear away:

'Thank you for putting your dish in the dishwasher without being asked.'

By involving your children at a family meal, you will be creating a sense of connection and providing a safe, informal place for them to share their thoughts and build supportive relations at home, which in turn will build their resilience and confidence going forwards.

Why boundaries matter

When eating together becomes more familiar and everyone is enjoying the interaction, it's time to start introducing a few boundaries. Establishing 'limits' forms the crucial second part of a truly effective parenting strategy.

First, it is good to be clear about what is expected at mealtimes. Gentle boundaries will make the experience flow more smoothly. Children need the structure of rules and consistent boundaries, even if they don't particularly like them. They tend to be calmer and more secure when they know what is expected of them. For instance, you might want to introduce the idea of everyone helping to clear up after the meal. Aim to give each child (and your partner) a particular responsibility. Younger children can help to create place cards or decorative menu boards for a special family meal, and even a three-year-old can help by carrying a plate to the sink, putting forks in the dishwasher or clearing things away. If you lavish enough praise on every offer of help you receive, you are likely to find children start to enjoy this responsibility.

By handing out tasks, you are not just sharing the load – you are teaching your children great habits about being a good family member and a thoughtful, considerate person, which will spill over to other aspects of their lives.

One important boundary is a screen ban: all phones and other screens should be turned off or at least put out of sight at mealtimes. And this should apply to everyone – adults included (children will copy what we do)! A TV or phones can very easily derail a family meal. Studies show that screens at mealtimes interrupt the hunger and feeling full cues, and children who use smartphones at mealtimes are more likely to be obese because the distraction makes them less tuned in to the tastes and feel of the foods, and less aware of how much they're eating. Keep a phone switched on and nearby only if you are expecting an urgent call or you need to check a fact that crops up in the conversation. Eating together should be a time to chat, enjoy the food and connect without other distractions.

Another 'limit' is serving one meal and only one meal for everyone and not falling into the trap of providing different meals to suit individual preferences. There will inevitably be grumbles, but if you lavish enough praise on a child for trying the tiniest taste of an unfamiliar food, they will eventually come back for more.

If someone does act up, don't engage. If your child is messing about, pay no attention. Talk enthusiastically among yourselves or focus on someone else at the table, as children don't like to be left out. Keep your cool and model the behaviour you want to see. Only engage when your child has abandoned the silly behaviour and keep a look out for better behaviour that you can praise. This should enable you to connect again. If anyone interrupts or misbehaves slightly, calmly say something to clarify what they have done ('We don't talk with our mouths full') and then, as soon as they comply, praise it ('That's lovely, you're eating really nicely now').

What's for dinner?

For the first few family meals don't worry too much about what you're eating. If you know you need to serve up pizza or burgers to tempt everyone to the table, that's absolutely fine. If things go well and the children enjoy eating together, you can gradually introduce the wonderfully healthy family meals in this book. You could start with some homemade burgers (see page 126) or firm favourites, like spaghetti Bolognese (see page 125) or Shepherd's Pie (see page 129). My recipes are surprisingly healthy because they incorporate hidden vegetables the kids might not even notice.

Once the idea of eating together becomes familiar – even enjoyable – you can gradually incorporate a wider variety of foods and, on some days, let the children choose the menu. It can really help if the children have been involved in the food preparation. The more they are part of the process, the more they can understand and appreciate the food that they are eating.

Some days you might try putting bowls of food on the table so everyone can serve themselves. This encourages independence and helps children learn portion control. It is also a great way to introduce new foods.

Another great switch-up is to get everyone to build their own meal – such as tacos, pizza or filled wholemeal wraps. You can all get involved in the preparation of the various elements (shredded lettuce, sliced peppers or capsicums, grated cheese, meat or fish, and so on), then lay everything out and invite everyone to dig in and create their own portion, encouraging them to take a little bit from each pile. Use as many tricks as you can to make eating fun – that might mean arranging portions into smiley faces, cutting bits into unusual shapes, or serving food in ways that make it seem inviting and colourful.

When introducing young children to new foods, it can help to limit portion sizes and choice at the table, so the process doesn't seem overwhelming. It may be easier to offer less and then add more if your child wants it.

Keep everything positive and praise your child for being adventurous and trying new things. Avoid bribery – it never works! By pressurising your child to eat a certain food, you could inadvertently be giving them the message that it isn't very nice and they only need to eat it under duress, which means it belongs in the 'yuk' category! Saying, 'If you eat all your vegetables, you can have a pudding,' puts pudding high in the charts and dumps vegetables at the bottom. Instead, be positive and open about all foods, commenting on how crunchy the apple is, or how sweet the carrot tastes. Talk about the food you're eating and take every opportunity to encourage positive attitudes towards it (see the table games on pages 38–9).

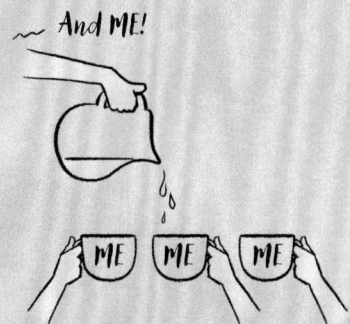

And ME!

ME ME ME

Table games

Playing silly games at the table during or after a meal can help with bonding and will encourage positive attitudes towards food and eating together. As mentioned before, it can also distract a fussy eater and move the focus away from potential food battles. Here are some of our favourite table games.

Food bingo
Create a simple bingo card for each meal with pictures of different foods (carrots, peas, rice, or chicken). When your child tries a food, they can mark it off. The goal is to get 'Bingo!' by the end of the meal, with small rewards, such as extra playtime or a sticker.

Taste test
Present different foods as a taste test challenge where your child guesses flavours or textures with their eyes closed. Use simple foods like apples, carrots and a sprinkle of cinnamon, to keep things familiar yet fun.

Food colour hunt
Pick a colour and challenge your child to find foods on their plate or around the table that match. For example, 'Find everything that's green,' which might include broccoli, peas or a green plate.

Crunchy or soft?
Help your child engage with their food by asking them to describe each bite. For example, they might say it is 'crunchy', 'soft', 'smooth' or 'chewy'. It also helps build their vocabulary.

Slip it into conversation
Give each child a word or phrase to slip into conversation during the meal without being caught out!

I spy
Play 'I Spy' using food items. 'I spy something red' could refer to a tomato or apple. This game keeps kids interested and engaged at the table.

Superpowers food game
Tell stories about the 'superpowers' of foods, like carrots giving night vision or broccoli making muscles strong, then encourage your child to take 'power bites' so they can activate their superpowers.

Who can chew slowest?
For a fast eater, challenge your child to chew slowly and enjoy each bite by seeing who can make their bite last the longest. This can encourage 'mindful eating'.

Tiny tastes starter
At the start of the meal offer small tastes of each food on the plate, and encourage your child to take 'tiny bites' or 'mouse nibbles' – this will make new foods less intimidating and can be quite entertaining.

Mystery plate

Create a small 'mystery plate' with tiny portions of one or two new or unfamiliar foods and ask your child to guess each food's name, or what it might taste like before trying it. This will turn trying new foods into a game and removes any pressure to finish.

Going on a picnic

Play this game by saying, 'I'm going on a picnic and I'm taking an apple,' then turn to the person on your right who repeats the sentence but uses a food beginning with 'b'. So, 'I'm going on a picnic and I'm taking a beetroot.' Keep going through the alphabet. For older children, you can increase the challenge by getting them to remember all the foods previously listed, in alphabetical order. So, 'I'm going on a picnic and I'm taking an apple, a beetroot, a carrot', and so on.

Conversation jar

Write funny or thought-provoking questions on little slips of paper, such as: 'Tell us about something you were grateful for today', 'If you had a superpower what would it be?', 'What's your favourite food?', 'What's your favourite animal and why?', 'Describe something you had to work really hard on' or 'If you were an animal, what would you be?' Put these in a conversation jar. If things go quiet at a meal you can pull out the jar and ask everyone at the table to take a slip and read it out. Or take the jar with you when you go out to eat – it should provide enough chatty distraction to keep the kids amused until the food arrives.

'Rose', 'thorn' or 'bud'

Everyone takes it in turns to be a 'rose' (they must say something funny or positive), a 'thorn' (they must say something difficult or challenging), or a 'bud' (they must say something they hope will happen tomorrow).

Roll an orange

Take an orange or a small ball to the table and explain the rules: whoever is holding the orange can talk. Once they have spoken, they must roll it to someone else. This is a clever way of slowing things down and giving each child a chance to talk and be listened to. It helps them learn the back and forth of taking turns and can also be a good way of calmly solving disagreements by making sure everyone has a chance to speak.

Conversation starters

Place an item of food on the table and ask: 'What could you make with this?' Or ask, 'Do you remember?' and invite everyone to talk about a memory they have. This is an opportunity to find out about family stories and share cherished memories.

Troubleshooting

Q: My children are so fussy – one won't eat potatoes, the other painstakingly picks out any onion! What can I do?
A: Most children go through phases of picky eating. One day they love carrots, and the next it's all 'yuck' and 'ugh!'. As frustrating as this may be, it's normal. Young children are naturally cautious about food. It is an evolutionary trait designed to protect them from eating poisonous berries or rotten food.

While some children will eat everything that's put in front of them, others will be less adventurous, may show strong preferences and will be hesitant towards both familiar and new foods. Children's food preferences are partly learned (they'll eat what they are familiar with eating and what they see others eating) and partly genetic. We know that some children can inherit a sensitivity to certain tastes (such as sweetness, sourness or bitterness) and textures ('slimy' foods like mushrooms and aubergine or eggplant can be tricky), while some might grow up to be 'super tasters', which means they actually have a greater quantity of taste buds on their tongue.

However, even the pickiest eaters can be persuaded to expand their food choices. Most children are able to adapt to different and stronger tastes and textures if you guide them with patience and lots of encouragement when they try new things. The key is to remain positive, calm and to continue doggedly to put the tricky or 'problem' foods in front of them. Studies show a four- or five-year-old child may need many exposures of a novel food to increase acceptance and it might take 15 or more attempts at tasting a new food before they become familiar enough with the taste and texture to accept it. You have to be prepared to play the long game!

Get into the habit of gently and persistently encouraging your child to try rejected foods at other meals alongside familiar 'safe foods' they are happy to eat. Seeing a food again and again should eventually help them feel comfortable enough to handle or taste it (and praise them enthusiastically when they do!). Avoid pressuring or bribing your child to eat a certain food, though, as this can make them even more likely to avoid it in future. Instead, try to offer new foods in a relaxed way and give lots of praise when your child is brave enough to try them.

It can sometimes help to tell your child all about the food they're eating. Show them the whole food first before chopping or cooking it. Encourage them to taste the vegetables or smell the fruit. While eating together, you can show your child how much you enjoy that particular food, and let the parental modelling trickle down. Talk about what you enjoy about it: its crunchiness, creaminess or juiciness. This shows a positive approach to food from which your child can learn. Children tend to imitate their parents during meals, so with time and repeated exposure, they're likely to become more comfortable with the foods when you eat together.

Q: I get so cross when my five-year-old messes around with her food and doesn't finish it. How do I avoid the daily battle?

A: It can be so aggravating when your children pick at the food you have lovingly cooked, moving things around on their plate – and you know only too well that they'll be complaining that they are hungry very soon afterwards.

Don't make it your problem. As parents, our job is to present the food and the children's job is to eat it. So, try to give the impression that the eating bit is not your issue, and remain calm.

Children's appetites vary significantly from one day to the next and, if you can keep a neutral atmosphere, your children will eventually learn that if they don't finish their meal, they may get hungry and they will have to wait for the next meal. It means you have to stick to your guns and keep the snack cupboard out of bounds, though, and certainly not accessible without your permission. Above all, avoid forcing a child to eat, or making them stay at the table until they finish. Better simply to remove the food after 20–30 minutes without a fuss and perhaps put a cover on their plate and tell them it is still there if they get hungry later.

Don't let food become your battleground, even if refusal feels like a rejection. Instead of resorting to bribery, focus on chatting at mealtimes, or even playing games (see pages 38–9), to move the focus from the food.

Q: My children are terrible snackers, helping themselves to the snack drawer whenever I'm not looking, and they aren't hungry when it comes to mealtimes. What can I do?
A: If your children have become used to grazing on snacks throughout the day, they might not be particularly hungry when they do sit down to eat. Grazing can make them more likely to turn their noses up at your home-cooked food (even though it is likely to be far more nutritious and satisfying than any factory-made, ultra-processed junk food).

Homemade healthy snacks (see pages 97–117) can be great fun to make together, and can provide a useful source of on-the-hop nutrients for young children. But be careful with your timings. It's a good idea to give children the opportunity to build up an appetite before your family meal, so they are more likely to eat what's put in front of them. Try using distraction (a quick game or a bit of drawing) to help your child learn to wait a little longer before eating, and praise them for waiting patiently. Slowly increase the interval they are expected to wait (and keep praising them for doing so).

Q: I'm worried that my son's weight seems to be creeping up. How do I keep his weight down while including him in family meals and not putting him on a diet?
A: If your child is a big eater and you're concerned that they might be eating too much, it is good to know that eating together as a family can offer protection against obesity, partly because family meals tend to be healthier, and partly because eating together tends to mean others are modelling healthy eating behaviours. In addition, children are more likely to eat more slowly while they are chatting, which gives more time for hunger cues to kick in and tell them they've had enough to eat. But that only works if you serve up proper home-cooked food and keep a close eye on portion sizes. Try downsizing your plates, bowls, glasses, mugs and serving dishes. Children don't need adult-sized

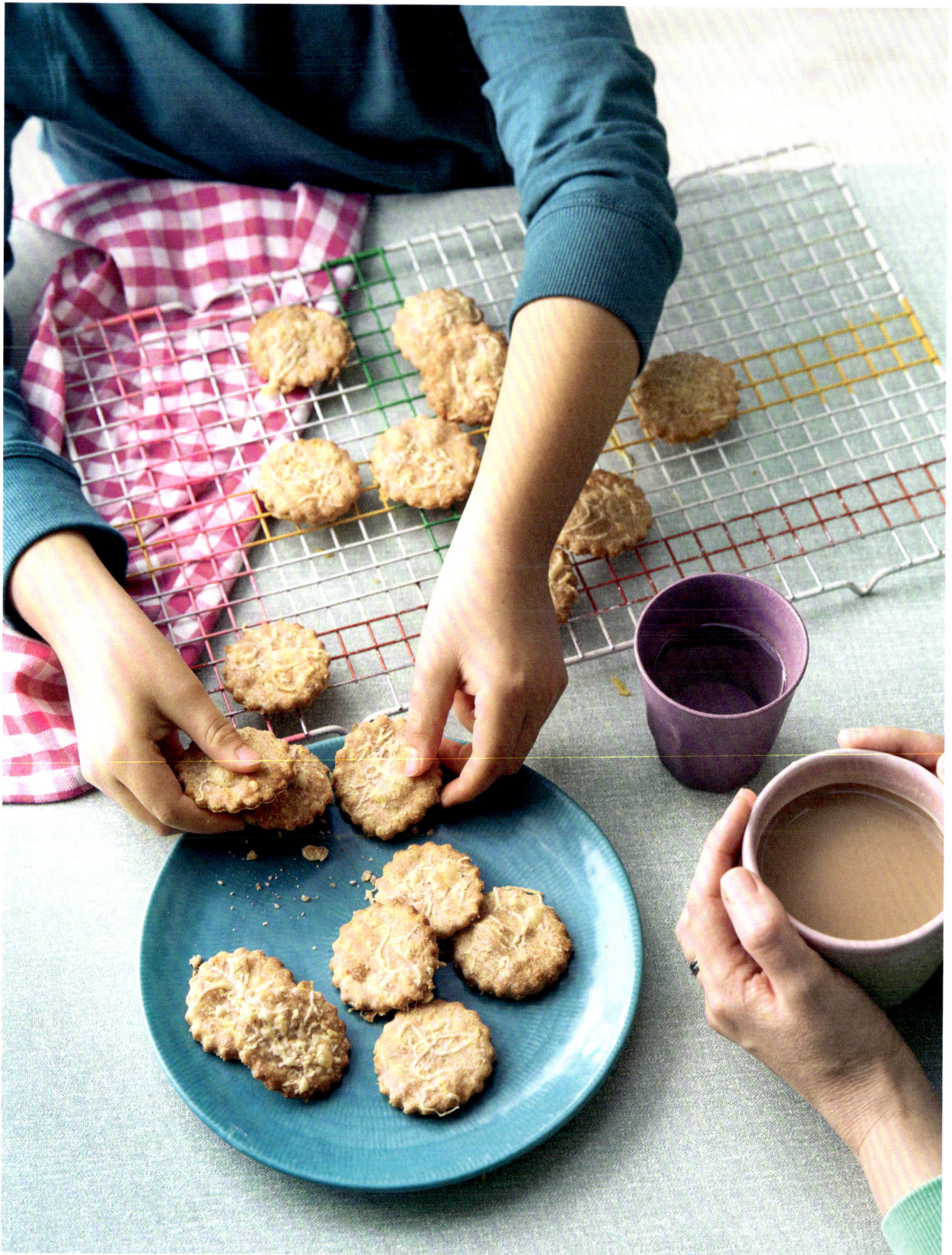

portions and studies show that, when they eat off smaller dishes, kids don't end up feeling hungrier, taking extra helpings, or compensating for eating less at one meal by eating more at the next.

Another tip is to plate-up in the kitchen and only bring the bowl of vegetables or salad to the table for everyone to help themselves to throughout the meal.

Don't talk in a critical way about your own body or your child's body, and make a point of encouraging and praising healthy choices, rather than focusing on weight, blame or dietary restrictions.

Remember that willpower is overrated and in short supply, so keep tempting foods and treats out of sight and try to reduce grazing, aiming to eat only at the table. And if your children have to snack, have healthy options on hand: place fruit bowls on the counter and pre-chopped vegetables in the fridge for easy access.

Q: I would like to eat as a family, but my partner is rarely home from work in time. How can we start eating together?
A: Get your partner on your side by telling them about the benefits of eating together as a family. See if it might be possible for them to come home a little earlier just one day each week, then gradually push back the children's dinner time to make a family meal more feasible. As you get into the routine and start to see the benefits, everyone should come to savour eating together. The kids will probably love it, they will eat better, and there's the added bonus that you only need to make one meal!

If weekday evenings are impossible, though, you could try to find a way of making extra time for breakfast as an opportunity to catch up as a family. This might be more likely to happen if you get together the evening before to make overnight oats (see page 53).

Q: How can I make my partner more enthusiastic about the idea of us all eating together?
A: Try using the sandwich technique: give a compliment or praise, express your concern/explain why you are so keen for this to happen, then give another compliment.

For example:

'The kids seem quite happy and settled; I think we are working well bringing them up together, don't you?' (Praise)

Then say:

'I'd love to have a chat with you about setting up regular family meals together, what do you think?'

If they seem reluctant, ask what their fears/concerns are. Perhaps they come home from work late, they feel too tired to face the children, or they don't want to eat 'kid's food'. Repeat those concerns back to them, to show you understand their reasoning. Then list your reasons for thinking that eating together is such a good idea. These could be: it brings you together as a family; it's a chance to get the kids involved in food prep; you'll only have one meal to prepare rather than two; you all get to practise listening and chatting, and this strengthens bonds; or studies show that families who eat together have children who are more likely to grow into better adjusted, more resilient adults.

Finally, address your partner's concerns point by point. If evenings are too busy, you could try the weekend. If they are reluctant to eat 'kid's food', you could train the kids to eat the same foods as you.

Finish the 'sandwich' by giving your partner another compliment or praise.

Aim to keep the conversation positive and upbeat. It can be hard for anyone to compromise and give ground if they feel their back is against the wall. Try to use 'I' statements rather than 'you' statements: 'I find it upsetting that the children are eating junk food', rather than, 'You encourage the kids to eat junk food.'

Q: My children are screen addicts and the only way I can persuade them to join us at the table is if they bring their iPads. What can I do?
A: It is important to understand just how addictive TV, phones and computers can be. We are biologically programmed to respond to visual cues in our environment – this is something that really lights up the brain, by bombarding its reward centres.

Screens can be a force for good – they can be a source of important information, and they can help children stay in touch with their friends, but they can overwhelm the brain in a very compulsive way. At times it may feel a bit like a pact you make with the devil, since they can be enormously useful as a way of occupying your child while you get on with essential tasks.

It is becoming increasingly clear, however, that we should be limiting our children's exposure to screens – for primary school age to under one hour a day rising to two hours a day at weekends. These are reasonable limits and children should be aware of the consequences if they overstep the boundaries. These consequences should be as immediate as possible and only last for a maximum of 24 hours. You might: turn off the wi-fi 30 minutes early; confiscate their phone for the evening; or cut their next playing time by half.

Start as you mean to go on by setting rules: decide what kind of screen exposure is okay for your household and write it down on a chart stuck on the fridge, or somewhere prominent. This could mean, for example, one hour a day of video games on Monday to Friday, but two hours a day at weekends. You might agree to stop screens two hours before bed time so they can have a calming wind-down routine to help them sleep. You might have a rule of no games until homework is done, which could save a lot of arguments, and your child should always have breaks during their game time. For example, every 25 minutes they should stop for 5 minutes and you should encourage them to do some physical activity.

Once you start enforcing these boundaries, the clear rule of no screens at mealtimes (unless mutually agreed to look up facts that have come up in conversation) should be easier to establish and adhere to.

Give lashings of praise whenever your child complies with the new regime. Don't just expect it, say things like, 'Well done for turning off your screen when we agreed', or, 'I noticed you stopped as soon as I asked.'

Dragging your children away from something so addictive may not be easy, but you will be surprised to discover how well children respond to praise and positive attention. If you are consistent, they will eventually learn to prefer that attention to the lure of their screens.

Recent research on 735 primary school children showed that children using their smartphones or screens at mealtimes were 15 per cent more likely to be overweight.

According to psychologist Dr Jonathan Haidt, there are concerns that screens are changing the way children's brains develop, too, affecting their ability to concentrate. This is clearly an area to keep abreast of.

Q: How do I persuade my teens that eating together as a family is 'cool'?
A: Teenagers are biologically driven to make a break for independence so getting them to the table can be a challenge. The truth is that teenagers think they don't need parental involvement but they do need a roof over their heads and good food. Although they may not admit it, they also need your nurturance and love. You can't force them to do anything, though – your best chance is if you can appeal to their better nature.

Start off by saying how proud you are of them, and because you appreciate their company, you would like them to join some family meals. Then ask them what they think about the idea of eating together as a family, listening very carefully and repeating back what they have said, to show that you understand their viewpoint. Be respectful, do not be sneery or snide, and avoid any temptation to add criticism to your tone of voice.

Next, expand further on why you think there would be benefits: 'It would be a chance for us all to talk together as a family', 'You will be able to hear from your brothers and sisters how they are getting on', 'Your little sister really looks up to you and I think she'd appreciate your views.' For extra weight, tell them that you feel quite strongly about the idea of eating together, that it matters a lot to you, and you would really appreciate it if they joined in. Say: 'I feel upset that I'm the one doing all the work

here. Let's talk about how many days a week you might be able to help me a bit – which evenings do you have a little more time? Would it be easier for you to help me with meals at the weekend?'

State clearly what you would like to happen and when, and ask them to consider being there. They may not be ready to give a snap answer and you may need to come back to the subject a day or two later.

You are more likely to be successful in getting teens on board if you can make the whole idea of family meals engaging and fun, and give everyone an individual sense of ownership around the meal – whether that's helping to plan the menu, choosing a favourite dish, or getting them involved in prep. Older teenagers can, with a bit of support, cook the entire meal themselves. It might oil the wheels if you invite one of their friends to join you, too.

Praise everyone involved for being helpful – praise goes such a long way.

Now you know what you should be doing it's time for the fun part – turn to the recipes in the second part of this book and tuck in!

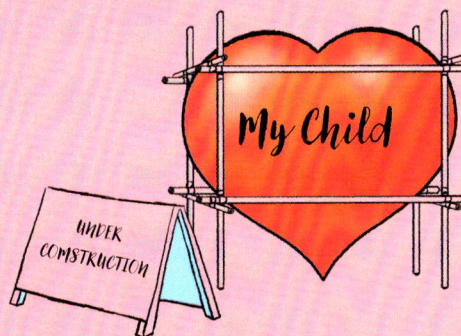

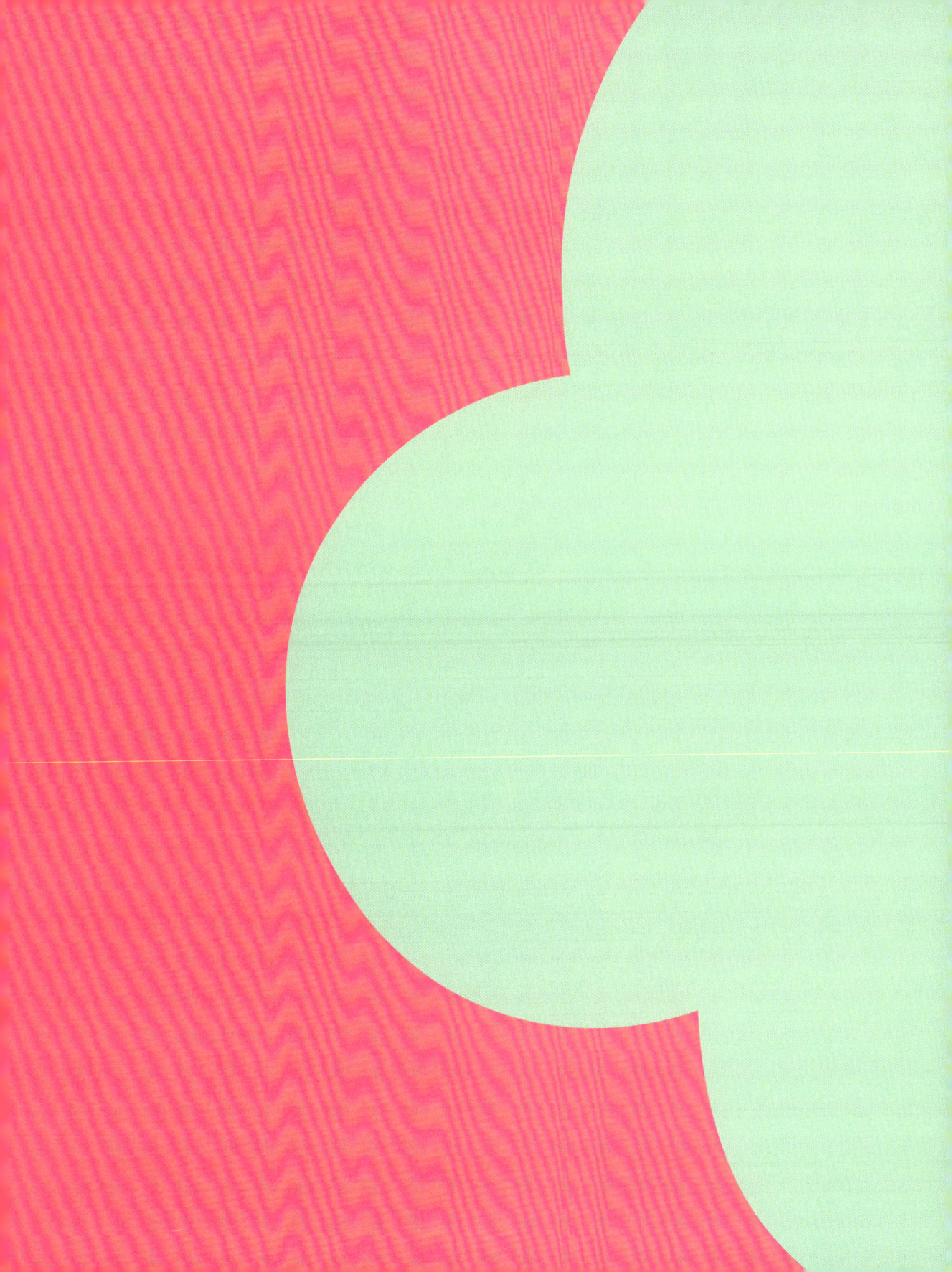

The recipes

This section of the book contains lots of fun, easy and nutritious recipes that your child can get involved in making – and then enjoy the fruits of their efforts – whether that means helping with our Make It Together Granola (see page 54), stirring the mixture for our Sweet Potato Hot Cross Brownies (see page 183) or, for an older child, cooking and building their own Lamb and Harissa Burgers (see page 126) with minimal support.

We hope you love the recipes and have fun in the process of cooking (and eating!) together with your child.

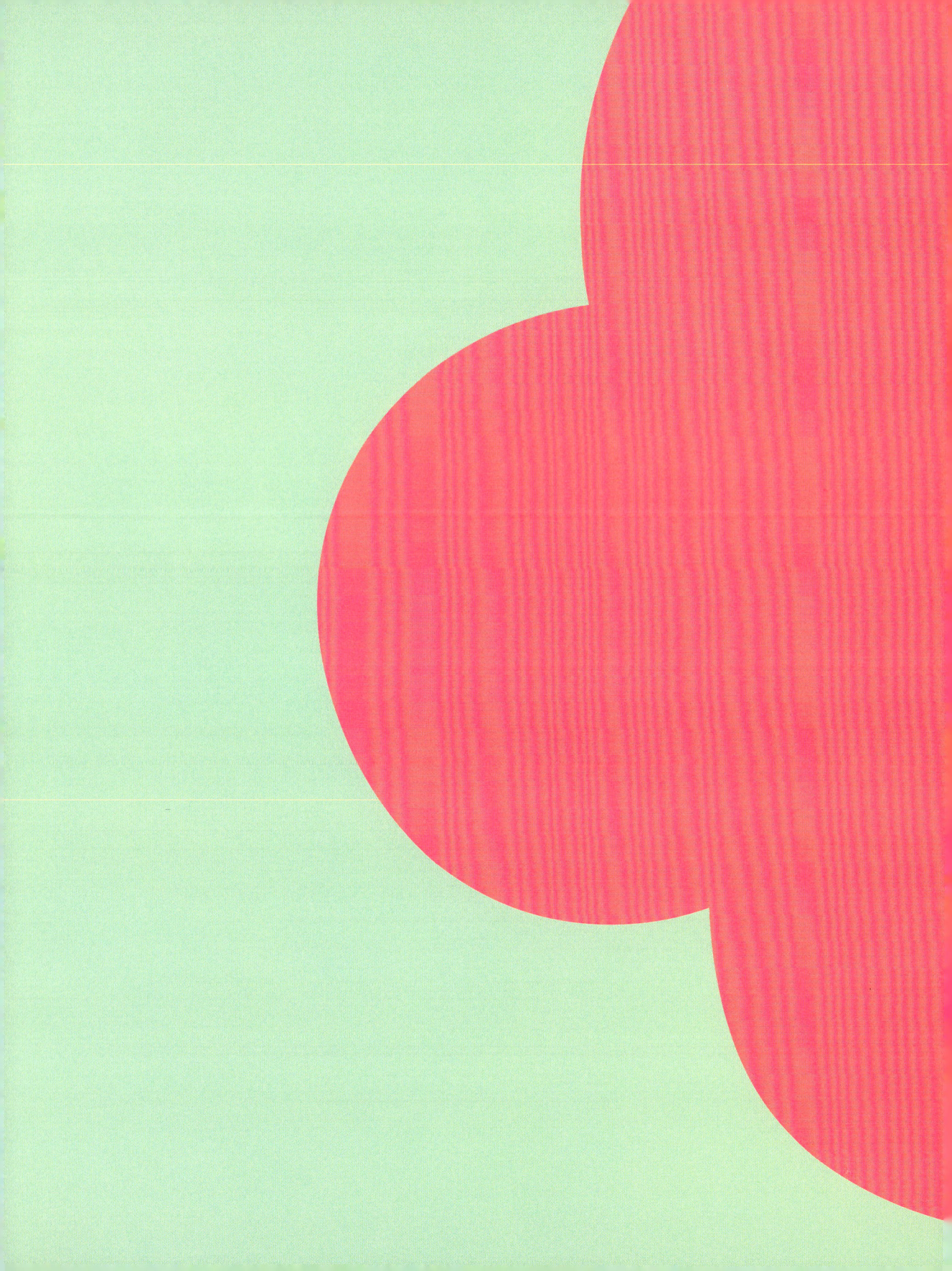

Breakfast

Strawberry Smoothie

This smoothie is somewhat like a milkshake and is a great way to start the day with some fermented food, thanks to live Greek yoghurt and kefir. The use of kefir and yoghurt introduces a wide variety of healthy bacteria into the gut, and children love to get involved when making this. You could also use it as a base for the Make It Together Granola (see page 54). Pour the thick smoothie into a bowl, as you would the yoghurt, and top with a few spoonfuls of granola.

Prep time 5 minutes | **Serves** 2

Ingredients
150g full-fat Greek yoghurt
100ml kefir (or milk of choice)
150g frozen strawberries
1 tsp maple syrup (optional)

Method
1. Place all the ingredients in a jug or deep bowl with a few cubes of ice and use a stick blender to blitz until smooth.
2. Serve immediately.

You can also freeze the mixture in ice-lolly moulds for a delicious dessert.

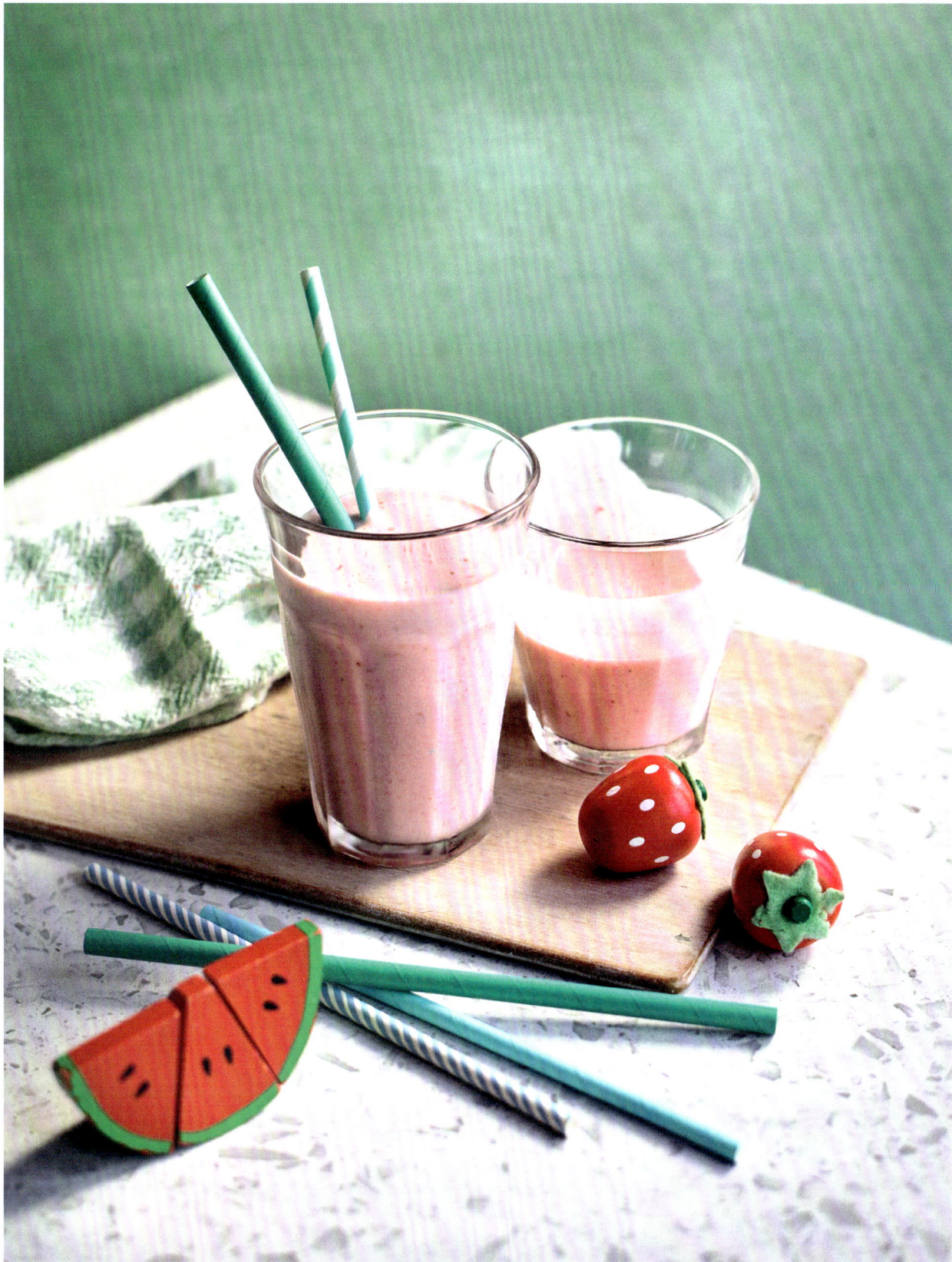

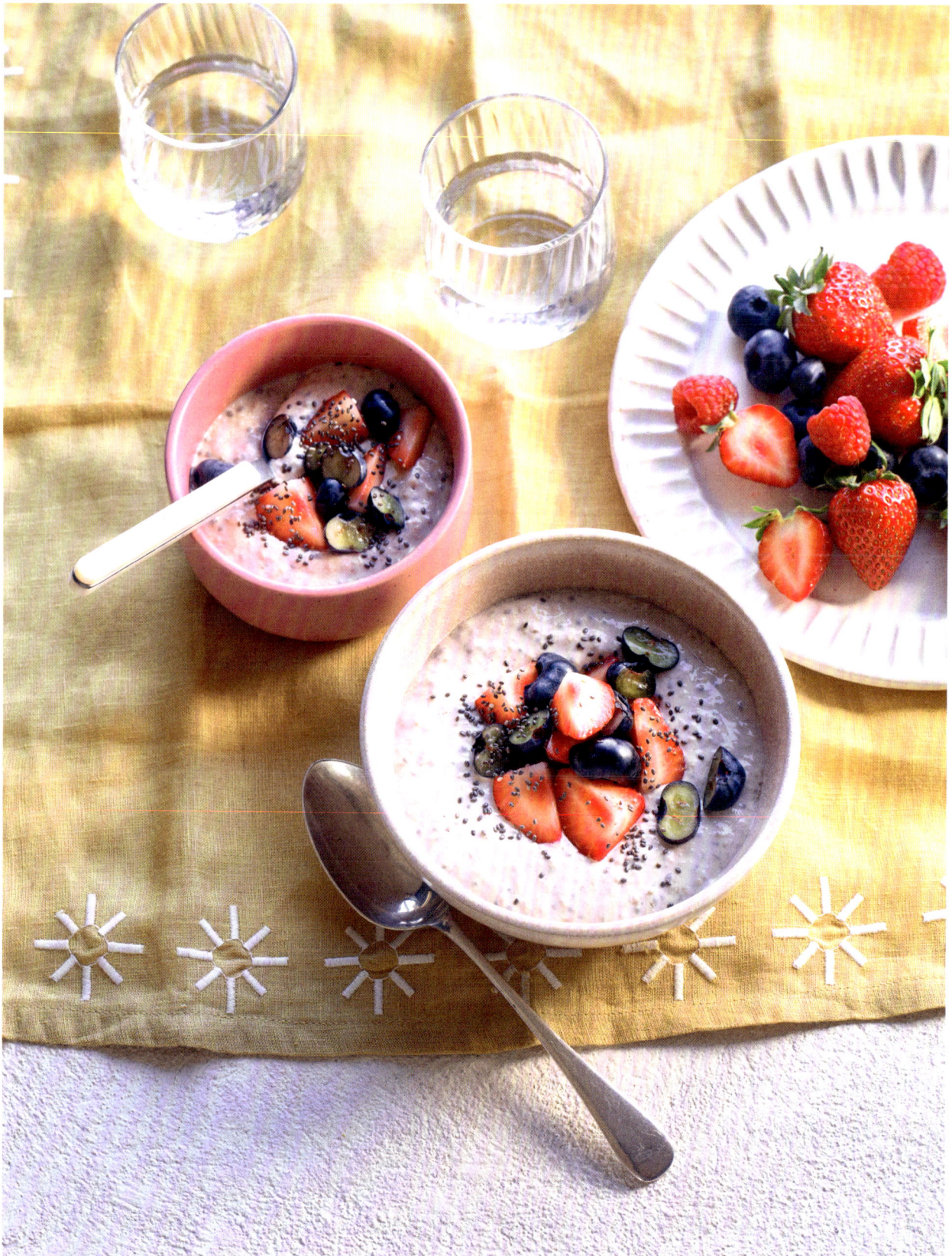

Easy Overnight Oats

Get ahead on busy mornings with these delicious overnight oats, with extra creaminess and fibre, thanks to the magic of the chia seeds.

Prep time 5 minutes, plus soaking time | **Serves** 2

Ingredients
1 small ripe banana
4 tbsp rolled oats (about 30g)
100ml milk of choice
100g full-fat Greek yoghurt
1 tsp chia seeds
½ tsp maple syrup (optional)
40g berries (such as blueberries, raspberries or strawberries)

Method
1. Put the banana in a mixing bowl and mash with a fork.
2. Add the oats, milk, yoghurt, chia seeds and maple syrup, if using, and mix to combine.
3. Divide between two bowls and place in the fridge overnight.
4. Top with the berries and an extra sprinkle of chia seeds before serving.

Make It Together Granola

Shop-bought granola can be laden with sugar, plus it's easier than you'd think to make your own. This recipe has only a small list of ingredients and would be straightforward to make even with children.

Prep time 8 minutes | **Cook time** 30–40 minutes | **Makes** 300g

Ingredients
200g rolled oats
100g flaked almonds
1½ tsp ground cinnamon
2 tsp vanilla extract
4 tbsp maple syrup
1 tbsp olive oil

Method
1. Preheat the oven to 150°C/Fan 130°C/Gas 2 and line a baking tray with non-stick baking paper.
2. In a bowl, combine all the ingredients and a good pinch of salt, and toss until the oats and almonds are thoroughly coated and moistened.
3. Spread the mixture out on the prepared baking tray and bake in the preheated oven for 30–40 minutes, tossing halfway through. It is ready when the oats are toasted and the almonds are golden.
4. Leave to cool, then store in an airtight container at room temperature.
5. Serve with Greek yoghurt and berries, or Chia Berry Jam (see page 174).

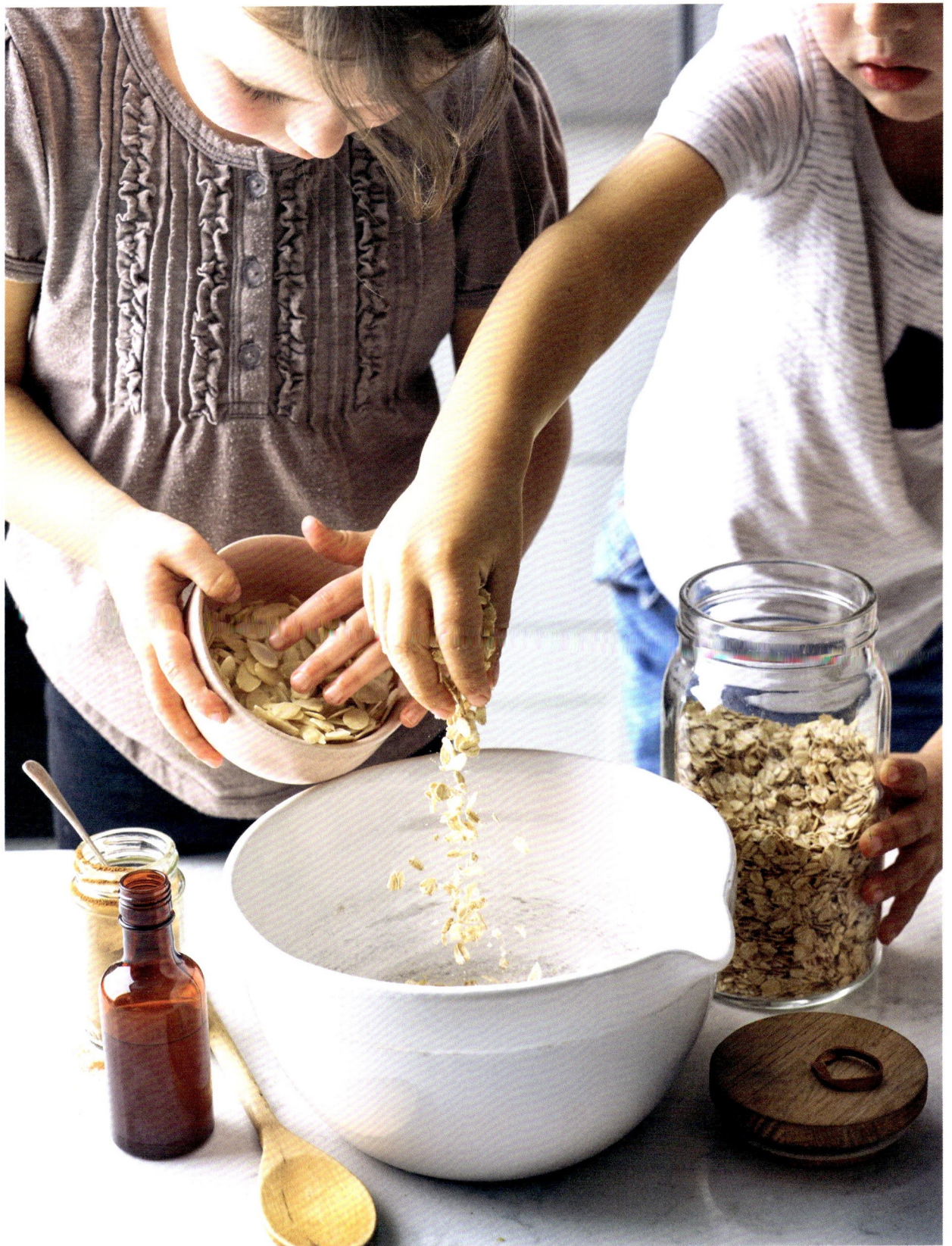

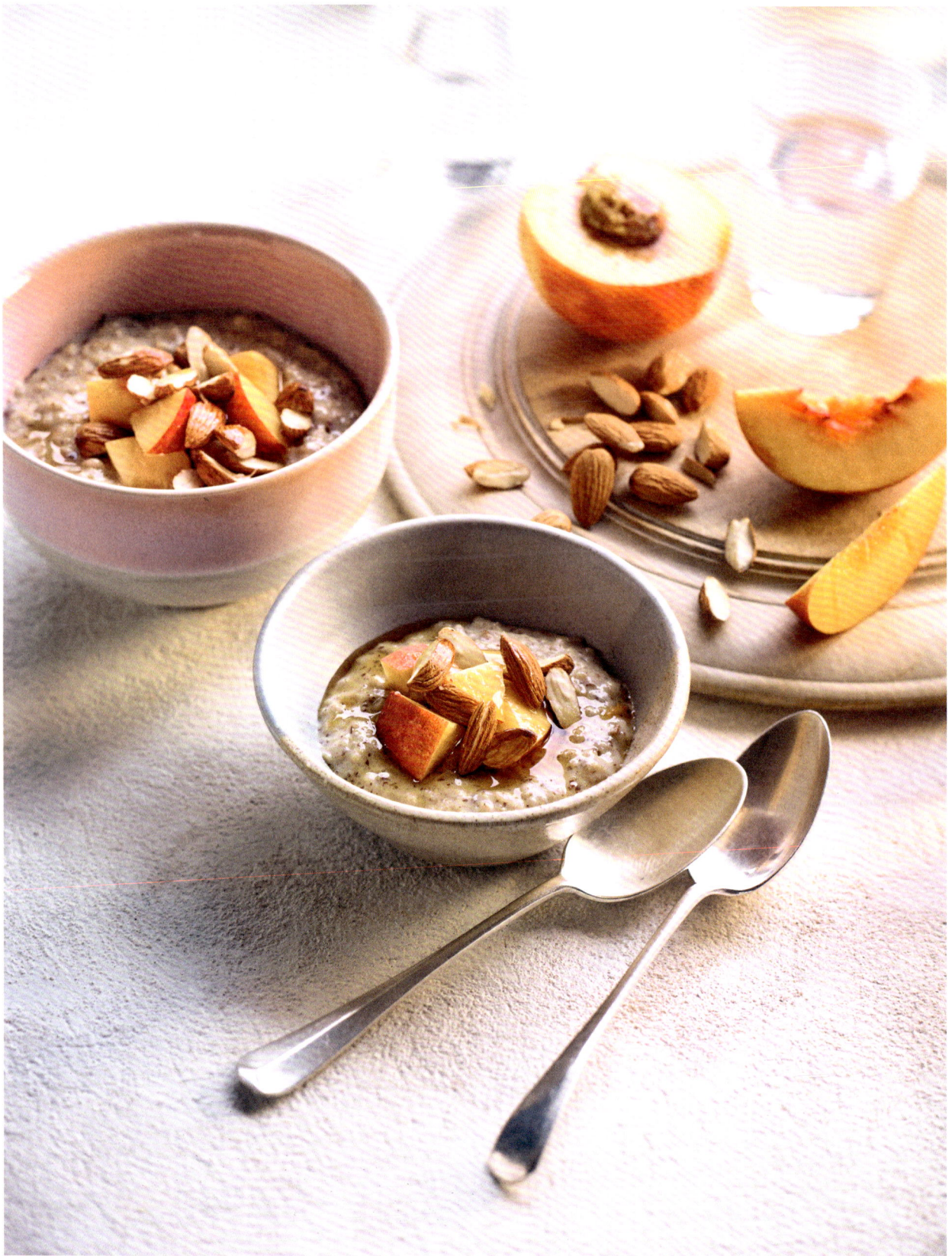

Turbocharged Porridge

Inspired by the flavour of caramel, this recipe contains high-fibre dates blitzed with milk and vanilla, and flaxseed added to the oats. The result is the creamiest, yummiest porridge you will ever eat.

Prep time 5 minutes | **Cook time** 6–7 minutes | **Serves** 2

Ingredients
300ml full-fat milk (or milk of choice)
3 soft pitted dates (about 30g)
½ tsp vanilla extract
60g rolled oats
1 tbsp ground flaxseed

Method
1. Place the milk, dates and vanilla extract in a non-stick saucepan and use a stick blender to blitz until smooth. There will be small pieces of finely chopped dates – this is okay.
2. Add the oats and ground flaxseed to the pan and place over a medium heat. Stir continuously for about 5 minutes until the milk comes to the boil. Once the milk is boiling, reduce the heat to low and leave to simmer for 1–2 minutes.
3. Divide between two bowls and serve with nuts and fruit, if you like, and a drizzle of maple syrup.

Strawberry Chia Pots

Strawberries are usually a real hit with children, and these Strawberry Chia Pots will be no exception. The recipe uses Strawberry Coulis, which is fun for kids to make. Along with being high in fibre, the chia also has an amazing ability to make food feel and taste creamy. It's fun to mix a teaspoon of chia in a cup and add a little water, stir it, and watch it become gooey!

Prep time 10 minutes, plus setting time | **Serves** 2

Ingredients
150g full-fat Greek yoghurt
½ portion (about 125ml) Strawberry Coulis (see page 177)
½ tsp honey or maple syrup
2 tbsp chia seeds
A few strawberries, to garnish

Method
1. In a bowl, mix together the yoghurt, coulis, honey or maple syrup and the chia seeds.
2. Divide between two small glasses and refrigerate overnight.
3. Top with strawberries to serve.

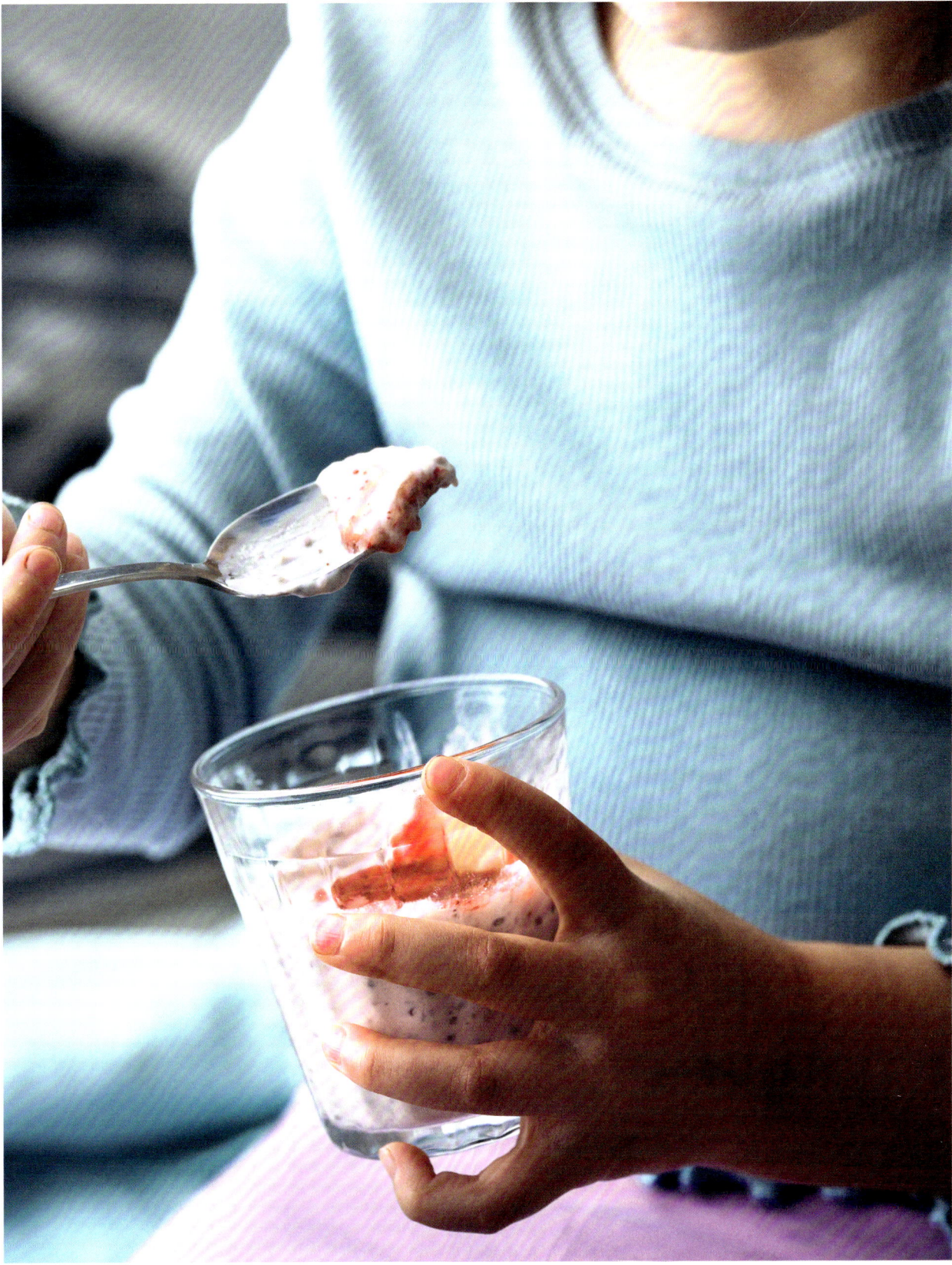

Chocolate Chia Pots with Raspberries

This creamy, chocolaty treat is wonderfully easy to assemble. Thanks to the magic of one of the superfoods, chia seeds, this will boost your fibre and protein, leaving you full for longer. It's also ideal as an overnight grab-and-go pot.

Prep time 10 minutes, plus setting time | **Serves** 2

Ingredients
1 tbsp unsweetened cocoa powder
150ml full-fat Greek yoghurt
2½ tbsp chia seeds (about 30g)
100ml milk of choice
2 tbsp maple syrup
70g raspberries

Method
1. In a bowl, mix the cocoa powder with the Greek yoghurt.
2. Add all the remaining ingredients, except the raspberries, mix again and leave to set in the fridge for about 4 hours, or overnight.
3. Top with the raspberries and a little extra yoghurt to serve.

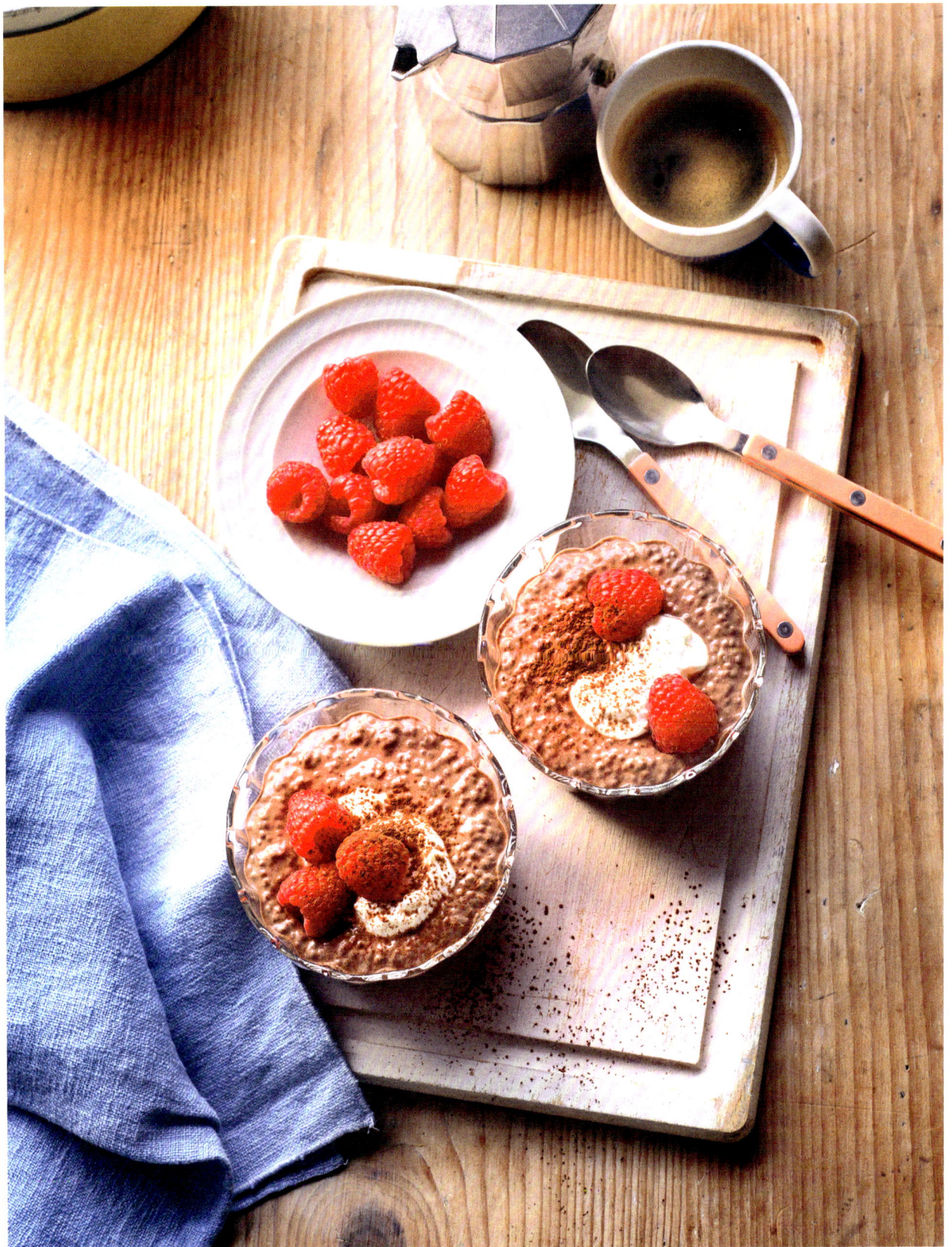

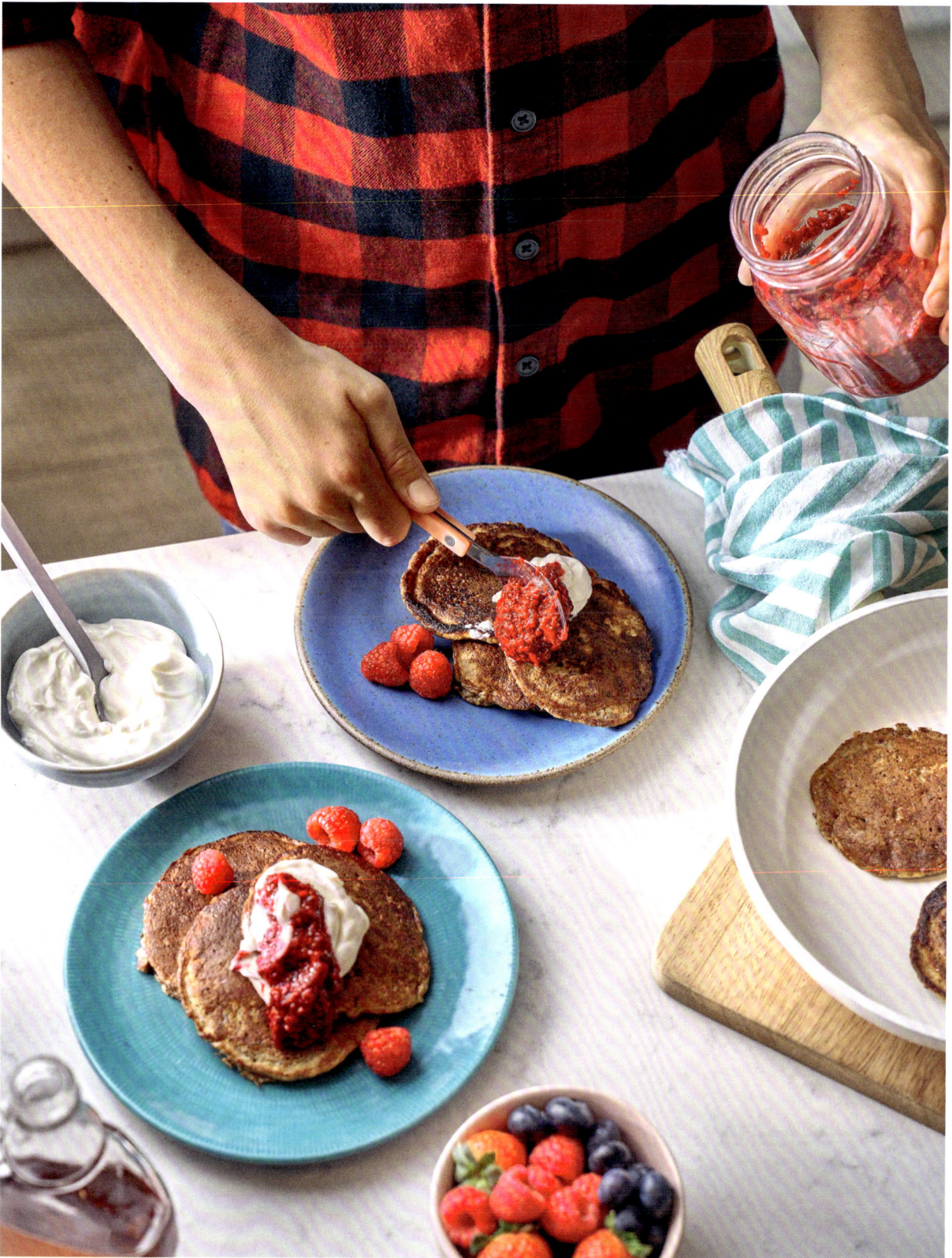

Apple and Cinnamon Pancakes

These pancakes are delicate in flavour, which makes introducing ground flaxseed, as a new ingredient, somewhat easier. Recipe writer Kathryn serves these pancakes with a Strawberry Smoothie (see page 50) alongside, as a real Friday treat in her household.

Prep time 5 minutes | **Cook time** 10 minutes | **Makes** 6

Ingredients
55g ground flaxseed
2 medium eggs
50ml milk of choice
1 tsp vanilla extract
1 tsp maple syrup
½ tsp baking powder
1 tsp ground cinnamon
1 medium red apple, cored and coarsely grated
2 tsp olive oil or butter

Method
1. In a bowl, combine all the ingredients except the olive oil or butter and whisk until smooth.
2. Heat 1 teaspoon of the oil or butter in a large frying pan set over a medium heat. Add 3 spoonfuls of the batter, spaced apart, and fry for 2–3 minutes. Carefully flip the pancakes and cook for 1 minute on the other side.
3. Repeat with the remaining oil and batter.
4. Eat the pancakes warm or leave them to cool and serve later as a cold snack. Try serving them with a teaspoon of Chia Berry Jam (see page 174), a few berries and some full-fat Greek yoghurt.

Chorizo and Tomato Scrambled Eggs

This is a classic, fuss-free recipe for scrambled eggs that will work every time. We have included some chorizo and tomato for added flavour and protein. For a quick and simple variation, skip the chorizo and go straight to step 2.

Prep time 5 minutes | **Cook time** 8 minutes | **Serves** 2

Ingredients
25g chorizo, finely chopped
1 medium tomato, finely chopped
4 medium eggs
2 slices of Spelt Soda Bread (see page 114) or bread of choice, toasted

Method
1. Place the chorizo in a small non-stick saucepan over a low heat and fry for 2 minutes. When it starts to release its oil, increase the heat to medium and fry for 1 minute until crispy. Add the tomato and cook for 1 minute, until the tomato softens a little. Remove the tomato and chorizo from the saucepan and set aside.
2. Take the pan off the heat and break in the eggs. Whisk the eggs, then return the pan to a very low heat and start stirring with a wooden spoon or spatula. Keep stirring all the time until the eggs begin to cook. Thick silky lumps will start to form as you stir. Carry on stirring until the eggs are ready – they should still be loose and moist. Immediately remove the pan from the heat or they will continue to cook.
3. Fold the chorizo and tomato into the scrambled eggs and serve on the toast.

Smoked salmon makes a nice substitute for chorizo here. Simply fry the chopped tomatoes in a little oil and fold into the scrambled eggs with some finely chopped salmon before serving.

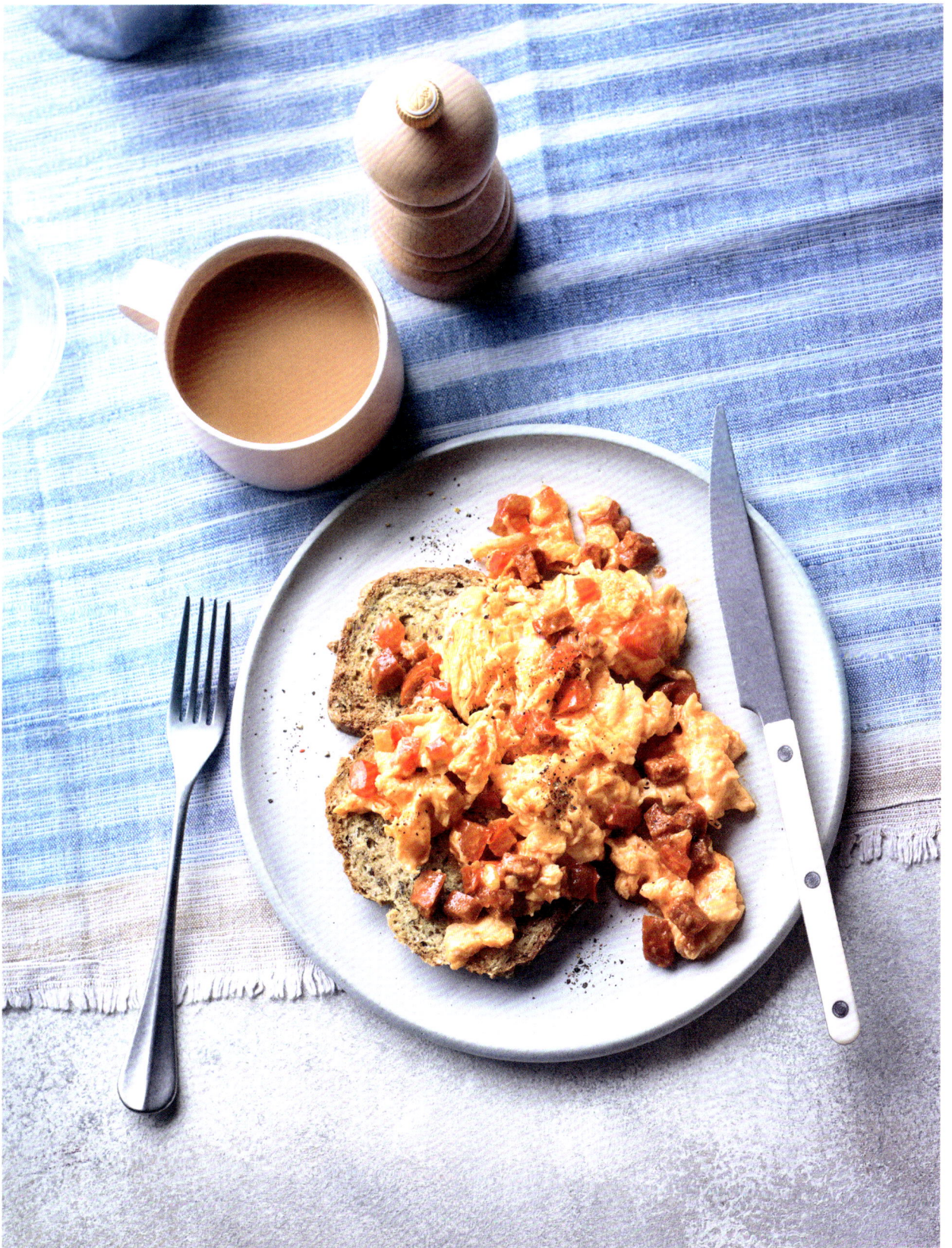

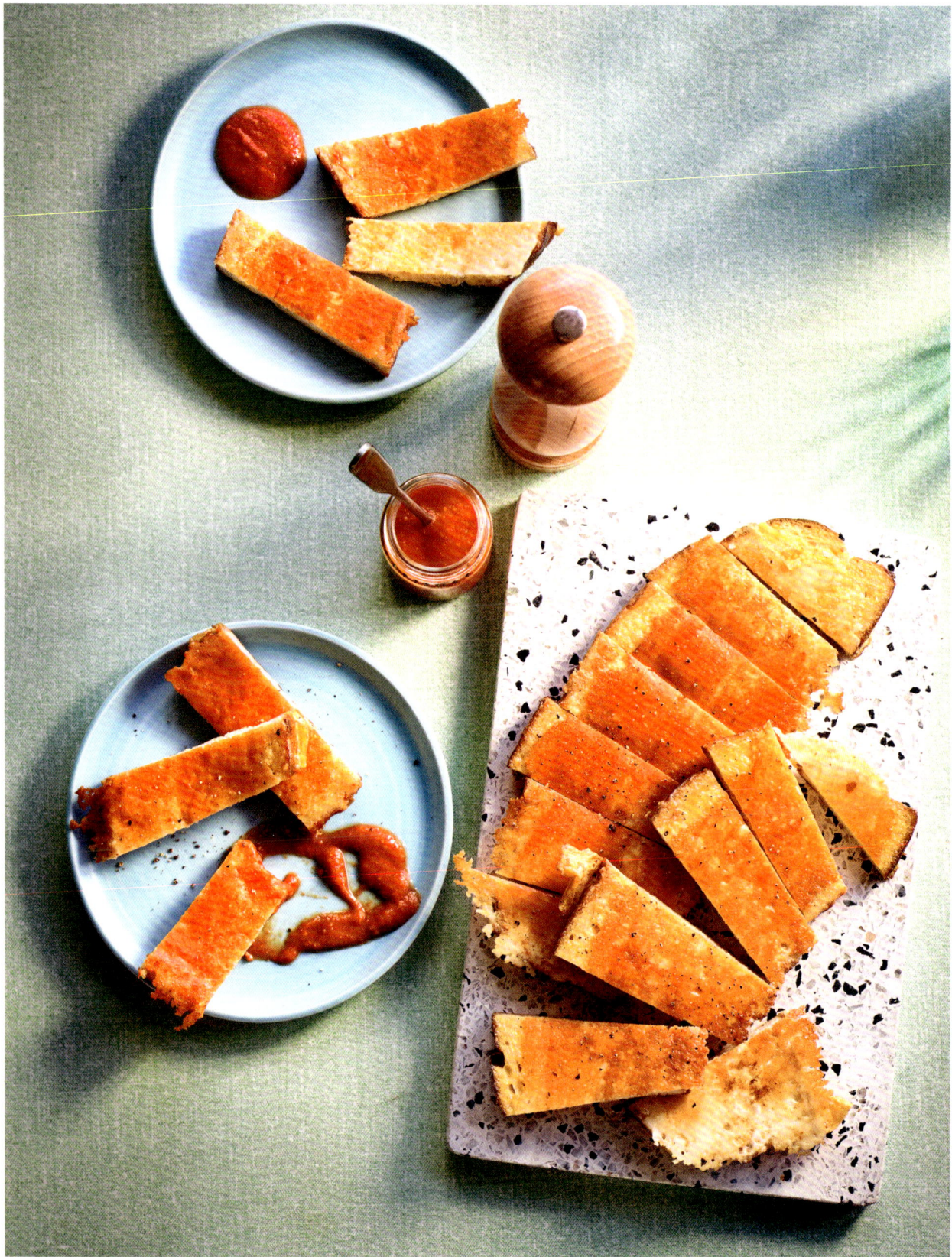

Eggy Bread with Cheese

This is a fabulous variation of a savoury breakfast – one that will keep you going well into lunchtime, thanks to all the protein to see you through the day.

Prep time 1 minute | **Cook time** 4 minutes | **Serves** 1

Ingredients
1 medium egg
1 slice of wholemeal or seeded sourdough bread
1 tsp butter or olive oil
1 thin slice of Cheddar

Method
1. Crack the egg into a wide bowl and whisk. Add the bread and turn to coat in the egg.
2. Place the butter or oil in a non-stick frying pan over a medium heat. When melted and bubbling, add the bread to the pan and top with the cheese. Cook for about 2 minutes, until the bread is starting to brown, then flip and cook on the other side for another 2 minutes, with the cheese face down.
3. When the cheese is starting to melt, remove the pan from the heat and set aside for 1 minute.
4. Carefully flip the eggy bread onto a plate, cheese side up. Season with a little black pepper and cut into slices to serve with a little Homemade Tomato Ketchup (see page 167).

Devilled Eggs

Boiled eggs are great for children, whether 'dippy eggs' with soldiers, or a simple egg mayo. Timings vary slightly depending on how you want the eggs cooked – once the water is boiling, cook them for 6 minutes for soft, oozing yolks, or 7 minutes for a slightly firmer yolk, which is better for these Devilled Eggs. The name 'devilled' refers to the fact that they are a little bit spicy.

Prep time 5 minutes | **Cook time** 7 minutes | **Serves** 1–2

Ingredients
2 medium eggs
½ tbsp good-quality mayonnaise
½ tsp paprika

Method
1. Bring a small saucepan of water to the boil. Once simmering, gently lower the eggs into the pan. It helps if you use a spoon to do this, to prevent the eggs from cracking when they hit the base of the pan. Simmer for 7 minutes.
2. Transfer the eggs to the sink and run under cold water to stop them from cooking further. Crack the shells and peel them carefully.
3. Cut each egg in half, scoop out the yolk and mash this in a small bowl with the mayonnaise. Season the egg yolk mixture with a pinch of salt and freshly ground black pepper, then return some to the hole in each egg half.
4. Garnish with the paprika and serve with toast and Homemade Tomato Ketchup (see page 167).

Add a small piece of diced ham or smoked salmon on top for extra protein.

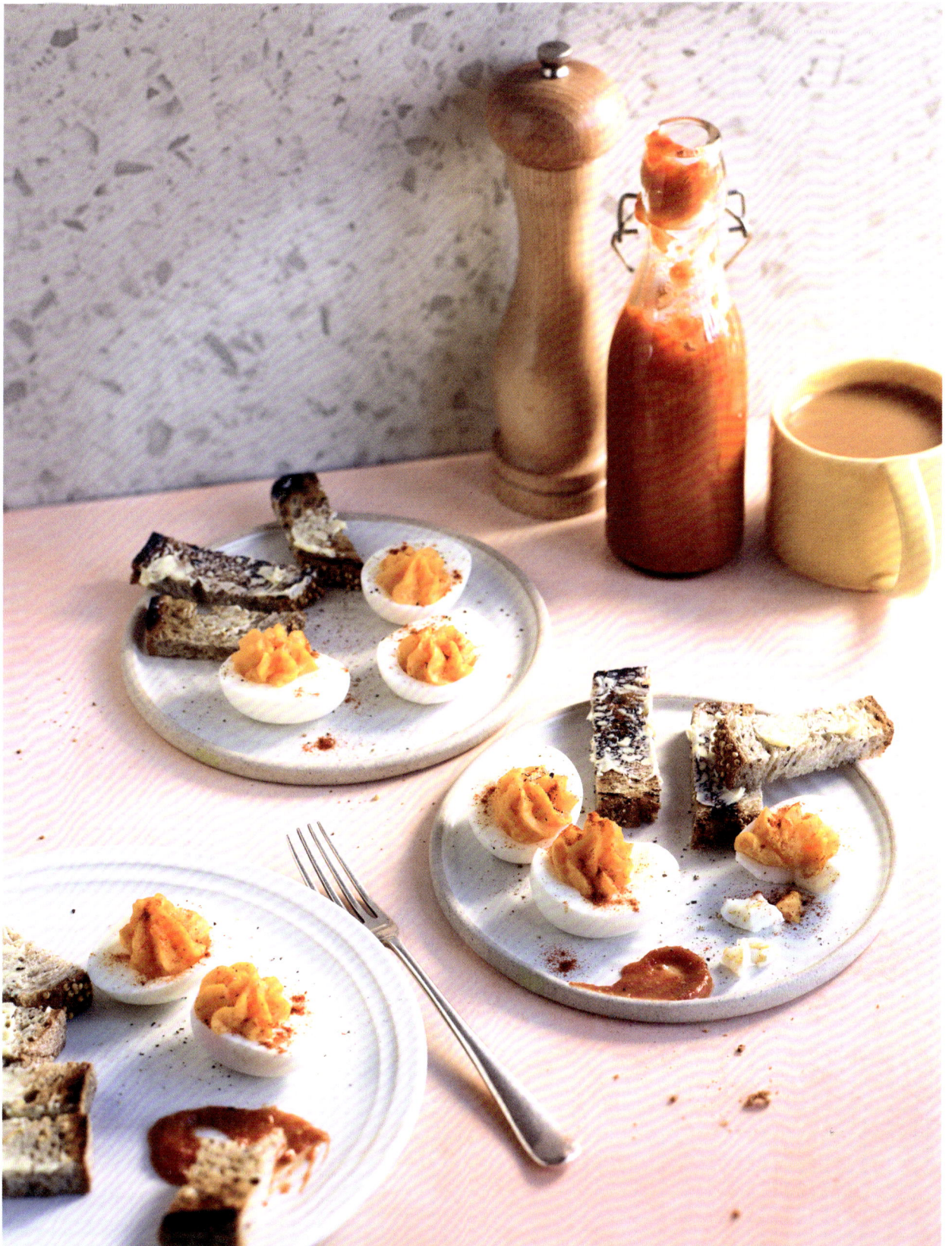

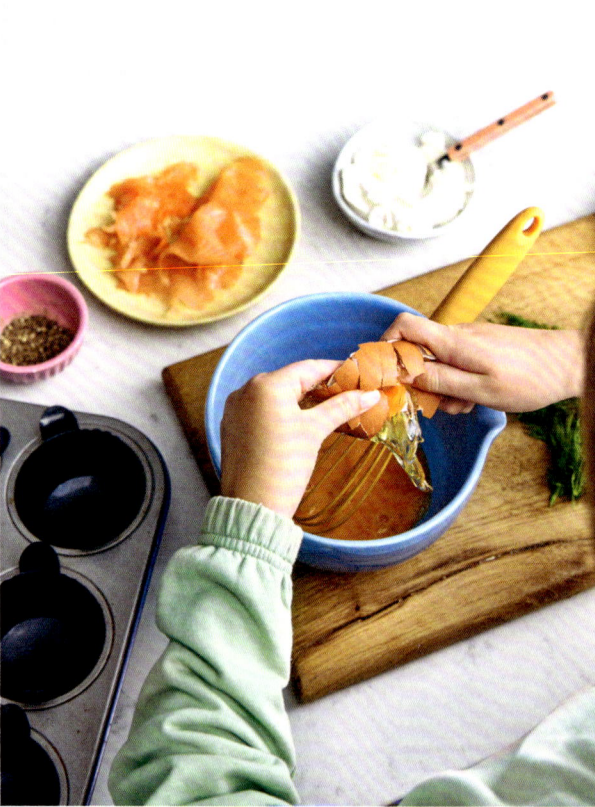

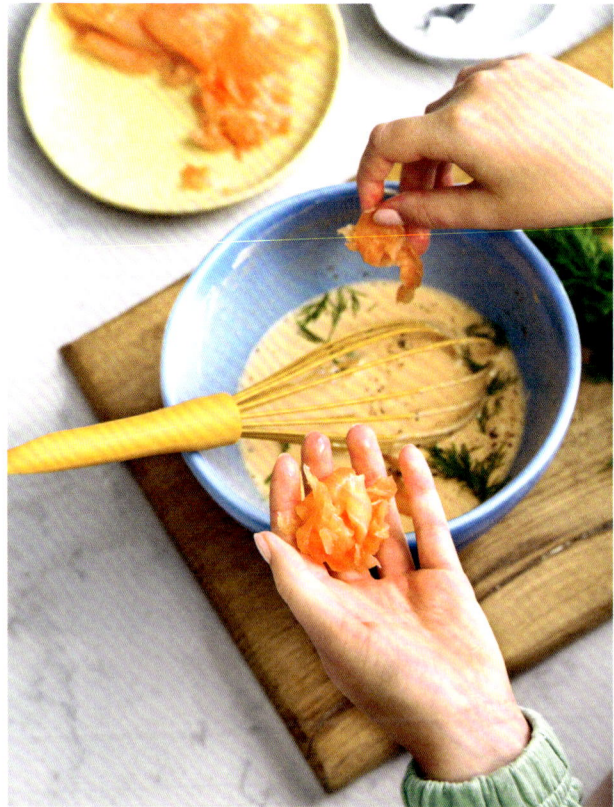

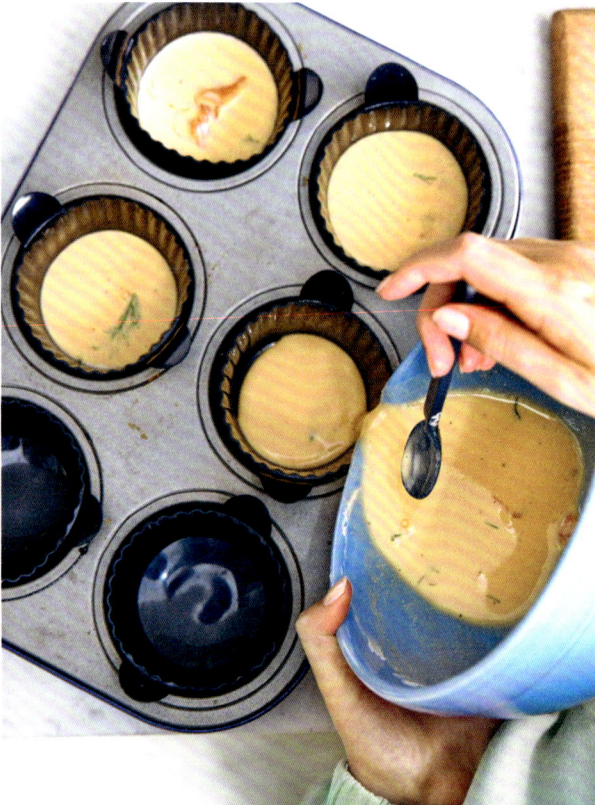

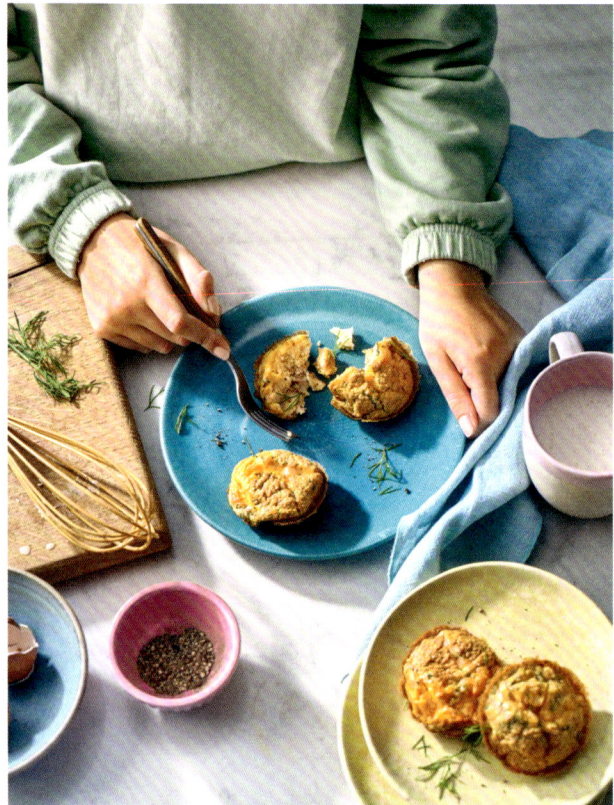

Salmon and Egg Muffins

Another brilliant savoury, protein-rich breakfast. Thanks to the salmon, you also get a top up of omega-3, which most of us are lacking. It's particularly important for growing brains. To top up further, chop up a little nori seaweed and scatter it in the bowl at step 2. Seaweed and algae are an excellent source of omega-3.

Prep time 5 minutes | **Cook time** 15 minutes | **Makes** 6

Ingredients
4 medium eggs
3 tbsp full-fat cream cheese (about 60g)
60g smoked salmon, finely diced
A few chives or sprigs of dill, finely chopped (optional)

Method
1. Preheat the oven to 200°C/Fan 180°C/Gas 6 and line a muffin tin with six muffin cases (silicone if possible).
2. Place the eggs and cream cheese in a bowl and use a stick blender to blitz until smooth. Season with salt and freshly ground black pepper and add the chopped salmon and herbs, if using.
3. Divide the mixture between the muffin cases and bake in the preheated oven for 15 minutes, until set.
4. Serve warm or leave to cool completely on a wire rack and serve cold as a grab-and-go breakfast.

You can use 85g finely diced halloumi in place of smoked salmon here, if you prefer.

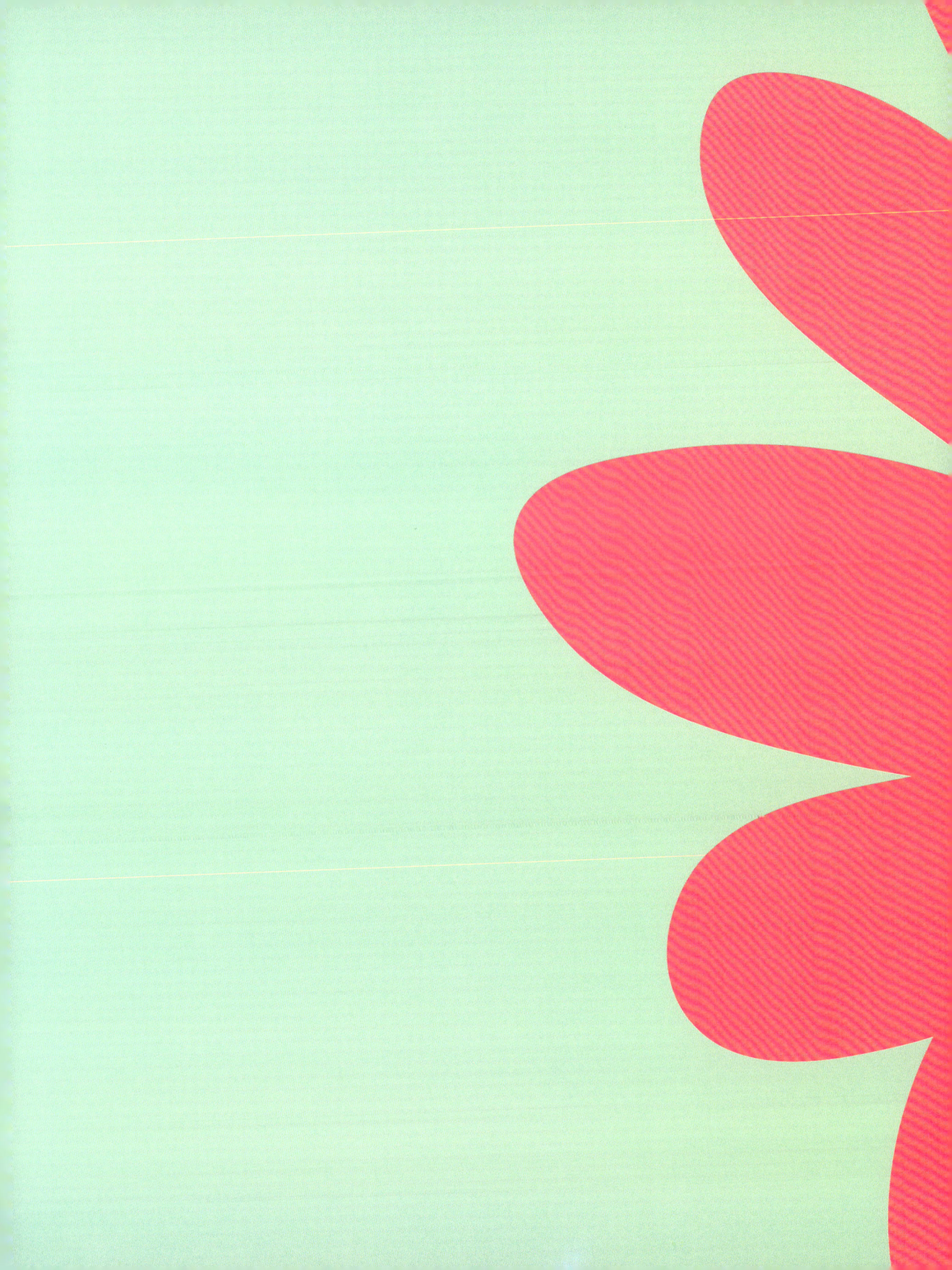

Lunch

Creamy Pea and Pesto Soup

This pea soup is lovely, soothing, comfort food. With the extra protein from the edamame and feta, it will set you up for the day!

Prep time 8 minutes | **Cook time** 20 minutes | **Serves** 4

Ingredients

1 medium onion, finely chopped
2 tbsp olive oil
150g frozen edamame beans
900ml vegetable or chicken stock
250g frozen peas
1 tbsp basil pesto
70g feta, crumbled (optional)

Method

1. Place the onion and olive oil in a saucepan over a medium heat and sauté for 3–4 minutes, until softened.
2. Add the edamame beans and stock and bring to the boil. Reduce the heat and simmer for 10 minutes.
3. Stir in the peas and cook for a further 5 minutes.
4. Add the pesto and remove from the heat. Leave to cool slightly then use a stick blender to blitz until smooth. The edamame beans will take longer to blitz than the peas, so persevere until you have a smooth consistency.
5. Season the soup with a pinch of salt and some freshly ground black pepper, and serve topped with the crumbled feta.

If you have fussy eaters, you can blitz the feta into the soup. Bear in mind that you may not need to add any extra salt if you do this.

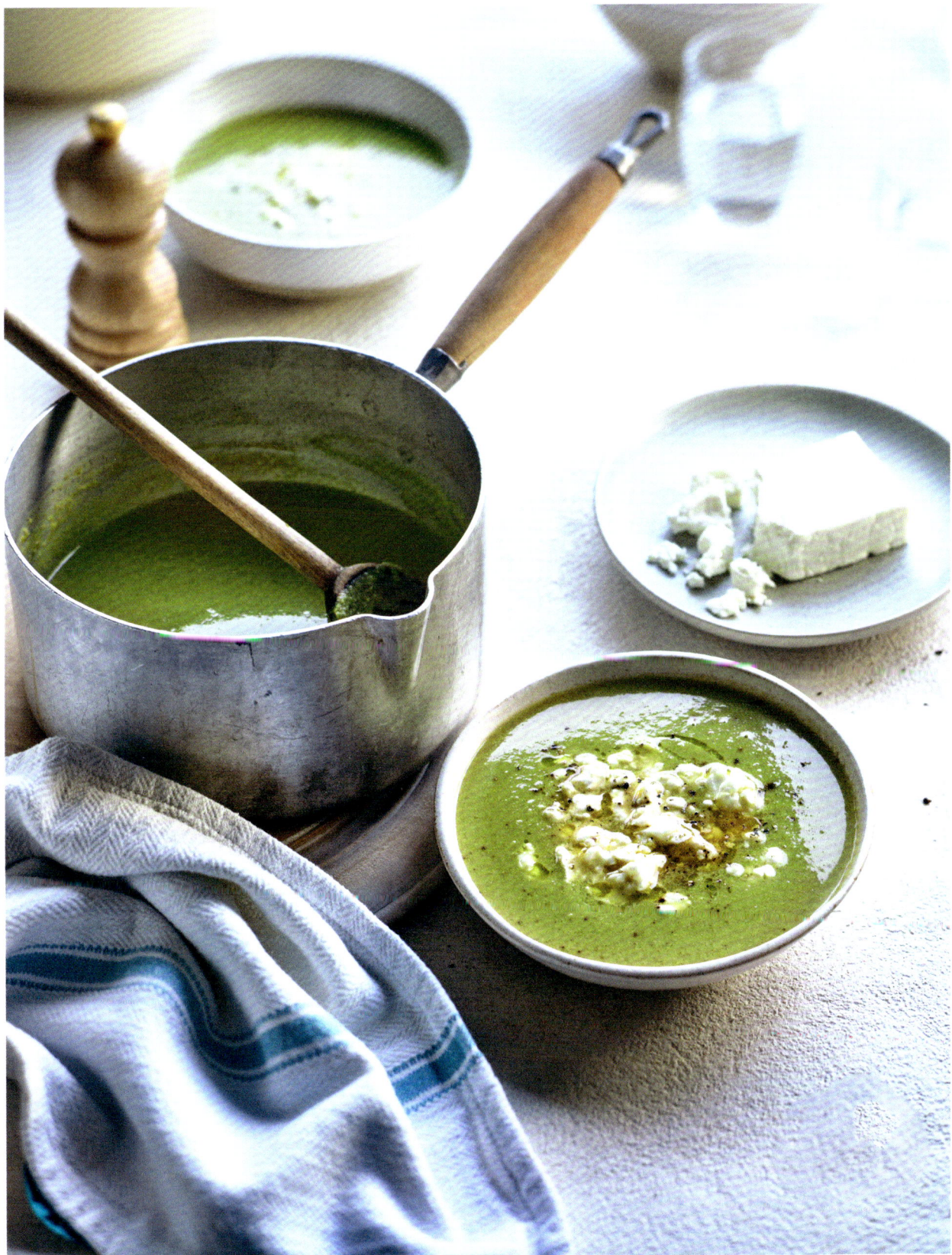

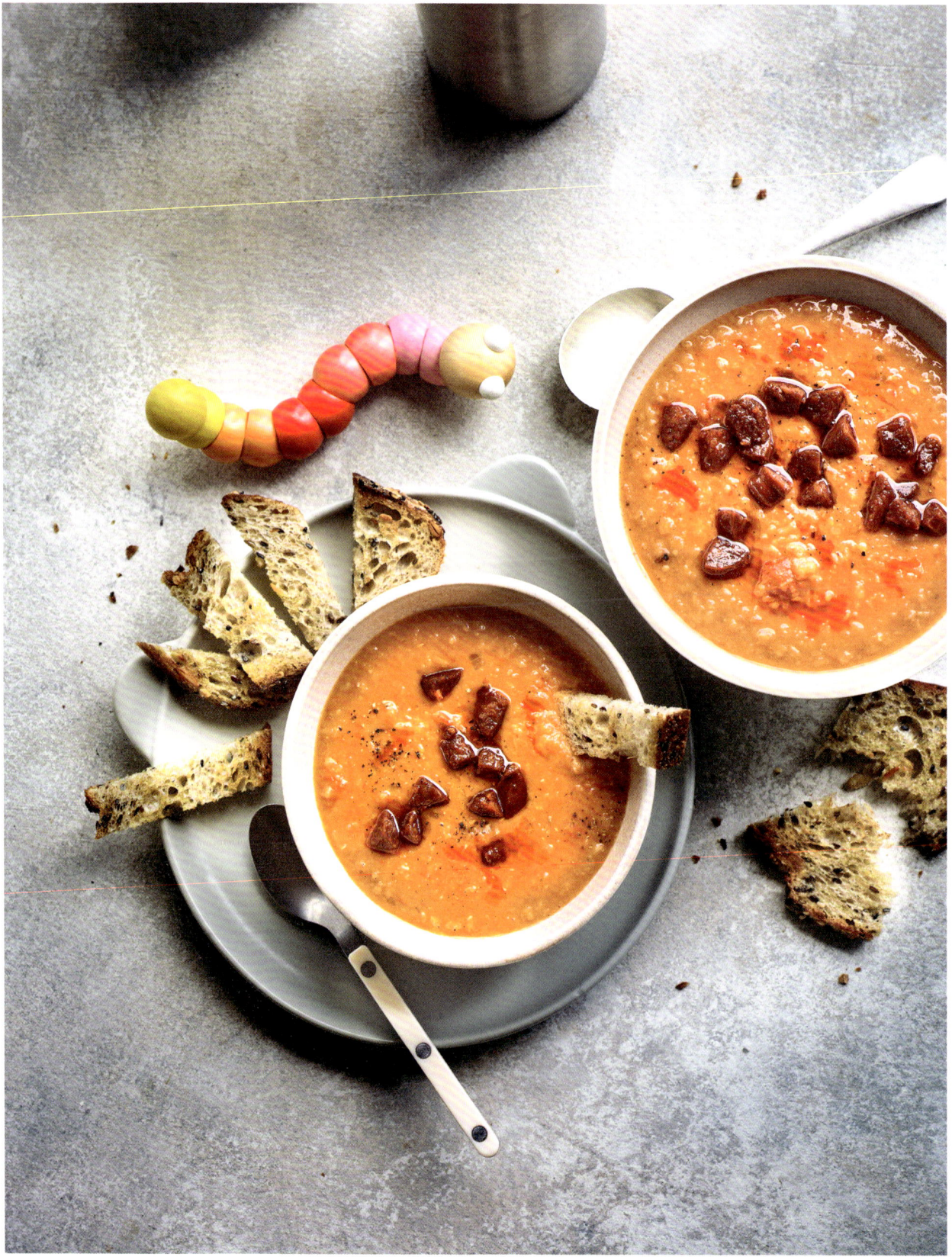

Lentil and Tomato Soup with Chorizo

Tomato is a flavour children are often familiar with, so adding lentils to this is an easy way to ramp up their fibre intake. You can omit the chorizo, if you wish – simply season the soup with paprika for added flavour and replace the chorizo with 85g diced halloumi. Fry the halloumi for a few minutes until golden and add to the soup before serving.

Prep time 10 minutes | **Cook time** 30 minutes | **Serves** 4

Ingredients

1 tsp olive oil
65g chorizo, diced (optional)
1 small onion, finely chopped
1 garlic clove, finely chopped
200g red split lentils
1 × 400g tin chopped tomatoes
1 vegetable or chicken stock cube

Method

1. Place the oil in a medium saucepan over a medium heat, add the chorizo and fry for 2–3 minutes until crispy, stirring all the time to stop it from catching and burning. Remove the chorizo with a slotted spoon and set aside, leaving the oil in the pan.
2. Add the onion to the pan and sauté for 3 minutes until softened. Stir in the garlic and cook for 1 minute more.
3. Add the lentils and stir to heat through. Pour in the chopped tomatoes. Refill the empty tin three times with water and add this to the pan. Crumble in the stock cube and bring the soup to the boil. Reduce the heat, cover with a lid and simmer for 20–25 minutes, until the lentils are soft and the soup is thick.
4. Remove the pan from the heat and use a stick blender to blitz the soup until almost smooth (or leave it chunky if you prefer). Serve topped with the crispy chorizo.

Tuna Sweetcorn Tarts

These tarts are a really fun recipe to make as a family – the children will love getting their hands messy and rolling out the pastry. Use the leftover pastry to make discs, cook them and sandwich two together with some Chia Berry Jam (see page 174) to make fun jammy dodgers.

Prep time 30 minutes, plus resting time | **Cook time** 15 minutes | **Makes** 6

Ingredients
50g salted butter, chilled and cut into 1cm cubes, plus extra for greasing
100g wholemeal spelt flour (or other wholemeal flour), plus extra for dusting
15g Cheddar, grated (about 1 tbsp)
1 medium egg yolk, whisked
1 × 125g tin tuna in oil, drained
½ × 198g tin sweetcorn, drained
3 tbsp good-quality mayonnaise
2 tbsp full-fat Greek yoghurt

Method
1. Grease six holes of a muffin tin with butter and dust with some flour.
2. Rub the butter and flour together in a large bowl with your fingertips until the mixture resembles fine breadcrumbs. Add the cheese and a pinch of salt and mix together. Add the egg yolk, along with 1½ tablespoons cold water. Bring the dough together with a blunt knife or fork.
3. Dust a clean surface with some flour and tip the dough out. Knead very gently to form a smooth ball. Dust with a little more flour and roll out to a disc with a diameter about 28cm. The pastry should be thin. Use a 9cm cookie cutter to cut out six discs and place them in the holes of the muffin tin, pressing down so the bases touch the bottom. Keep the leftover pastry to make biscuits (see above). Use a fork to pierce the base of each tart a few times and refrigerate for 10 minutes.
4. Preheat the oven to 200°C/Fan 180°C/Gas 6.
5. Bake the pastry cases in the preheated oven for 15 minutes, until golden and crisp. Set aside to cool.
6. Mix the tuna, sweetcorn, mayo and Greek yoghurt together in a small bowl and season with salt and a pinch of black pepper. Divide the tuna and sweetcorn mix between the pastry cases and serve.

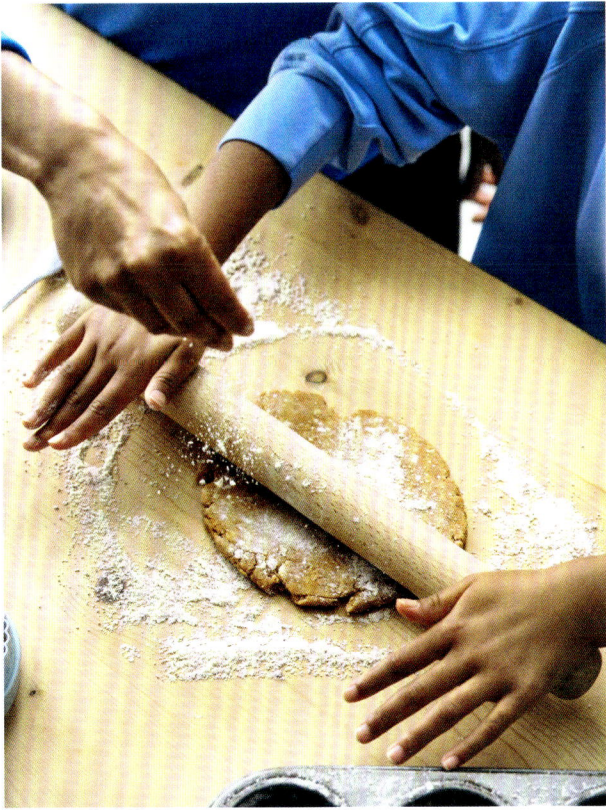

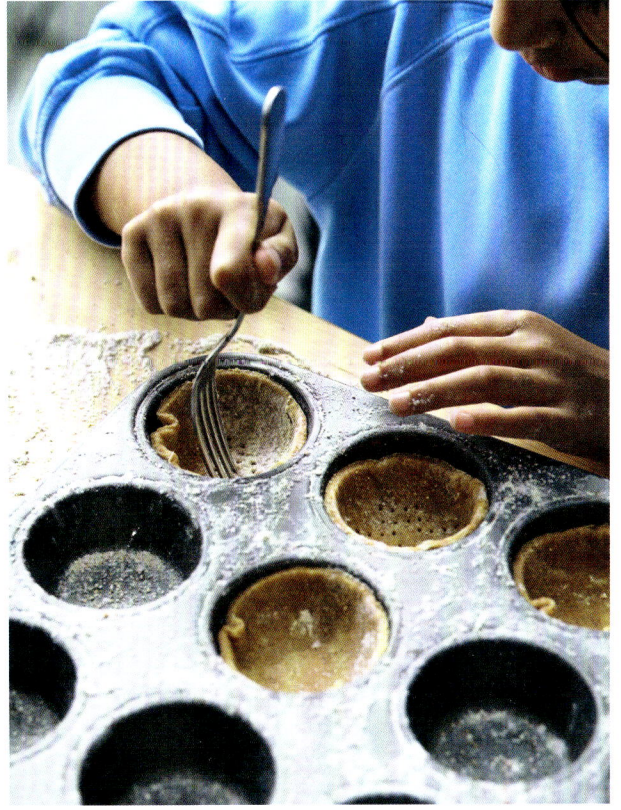

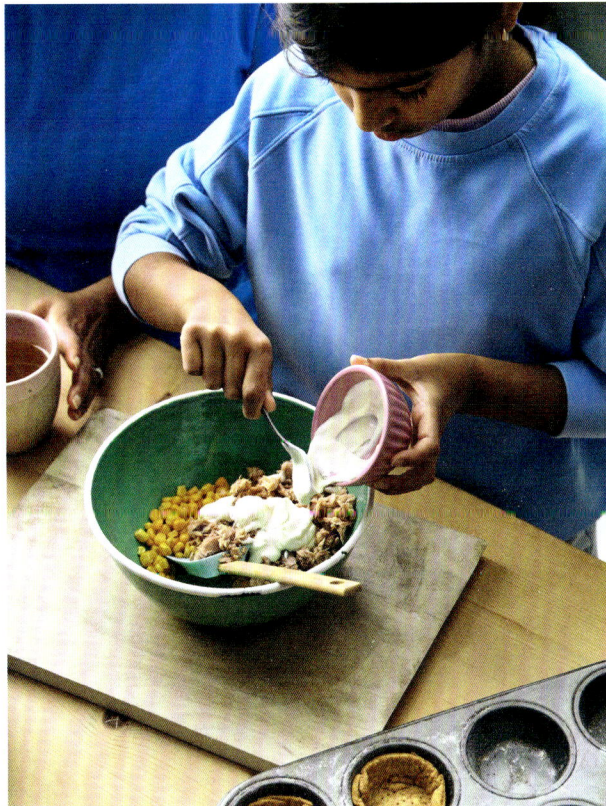

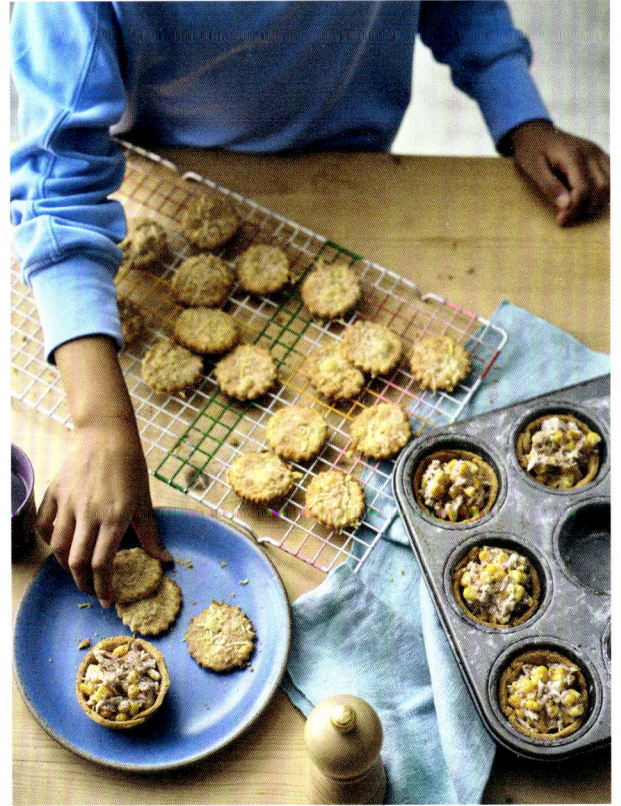

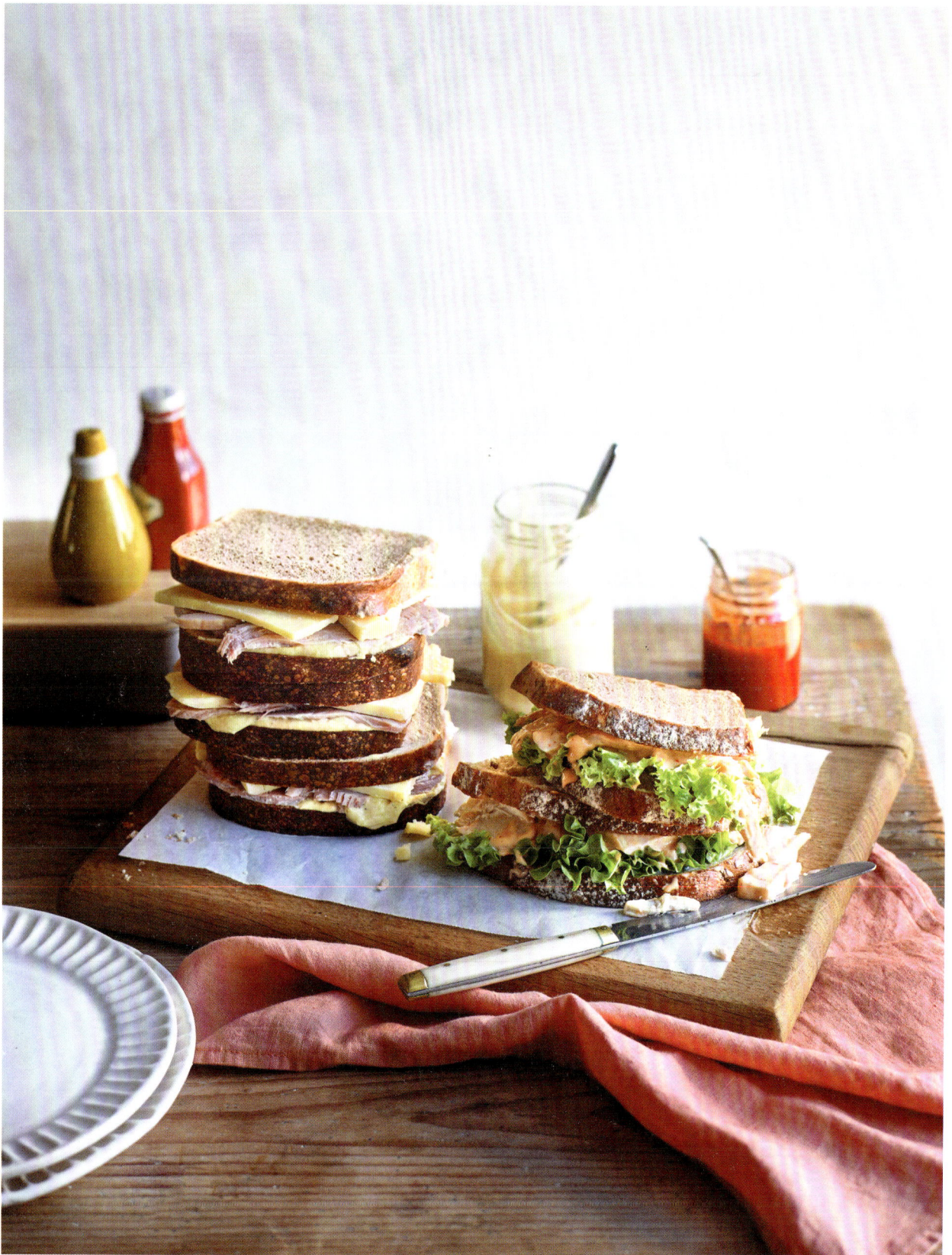

Two Easy Sandwiches

Leftover Chicken with Sriracha and Mayo

This first sandwich is a great choice for a lunchbox. Leftover cooked chicken provides an ideal protein boost and will keep you (or your child) well fuelled. Include some lettuce for added flavour and texture, if you like.

Prep time 5 minutes | **Serves 1**

Ingredients
150g leftover or shop-bought cooked chicken, roughly chopped
1½ tbsp mayonnaise
1 tsp sriracha
2 slices of sourdough, seeded or wholemeal, toasted if liked

Method
1. Place the chicken in a bowl with the mayonnaise and sriracha. Mix well to coat the chicken. Season with salt and freshly ground black pepper.
2. Spread the chicken over a piece of bread or toast and place the other on top to make a sandwich

Hummus, Ham and Cheese

This is so simple to prepare, there is no excuse for your child not to make it themselves! This combination of flavours is also delicious as a toasted sandwich.

Prep time 5 minutes | **Serves 1**

Ingredients
1–2 tbsp hummus
2 slices of sourdough, seeded or wholemeal
2 slices of good-quality ham
2 slices of Cheddar

Method
1. Spread the hummus onto a slice of bread and top with ham and cheese.
2. Top with the other piece of bread to make a sandwich.

Green Protein Pots

These protein pots are like crustless quiches and are so delicious. They would also make a great breakfast and can be baked in silicone muffin cases for a grab-and-go snack (the muffins will keep in the fridge for up to 3 days).

Prep time 8 minutes | **Cook time** 25–30 minutes | **Serves** 4

Ingredients
1 tsp olive oil
4 medium eggs
200g courgette (zucchini), grated
100g broccoli, finely chopped
60g feta, crumbled

Method
1. Preheat the oven to 170°C/Fan 150°C/Gas 3½ and grease four 250ml ramekins with the olive oil.
2. Place the eggs, grated courgette (zucchini), broccoli and half the feta in a medium bowl and use a stick blender to blitz until finely chopped. Season with a pinch of salt and some freshly ground black pepper.
3. Divide between the prepared ramekins and sprinkle with the remaining feta. Bake in the preheated oven for 25–30 minutes, until puffed up and golden brown.
4. Leave to cool slightly before serving, or leave to cool completely and serve cold.

Cheddar can be used instead of feta, if preferred.

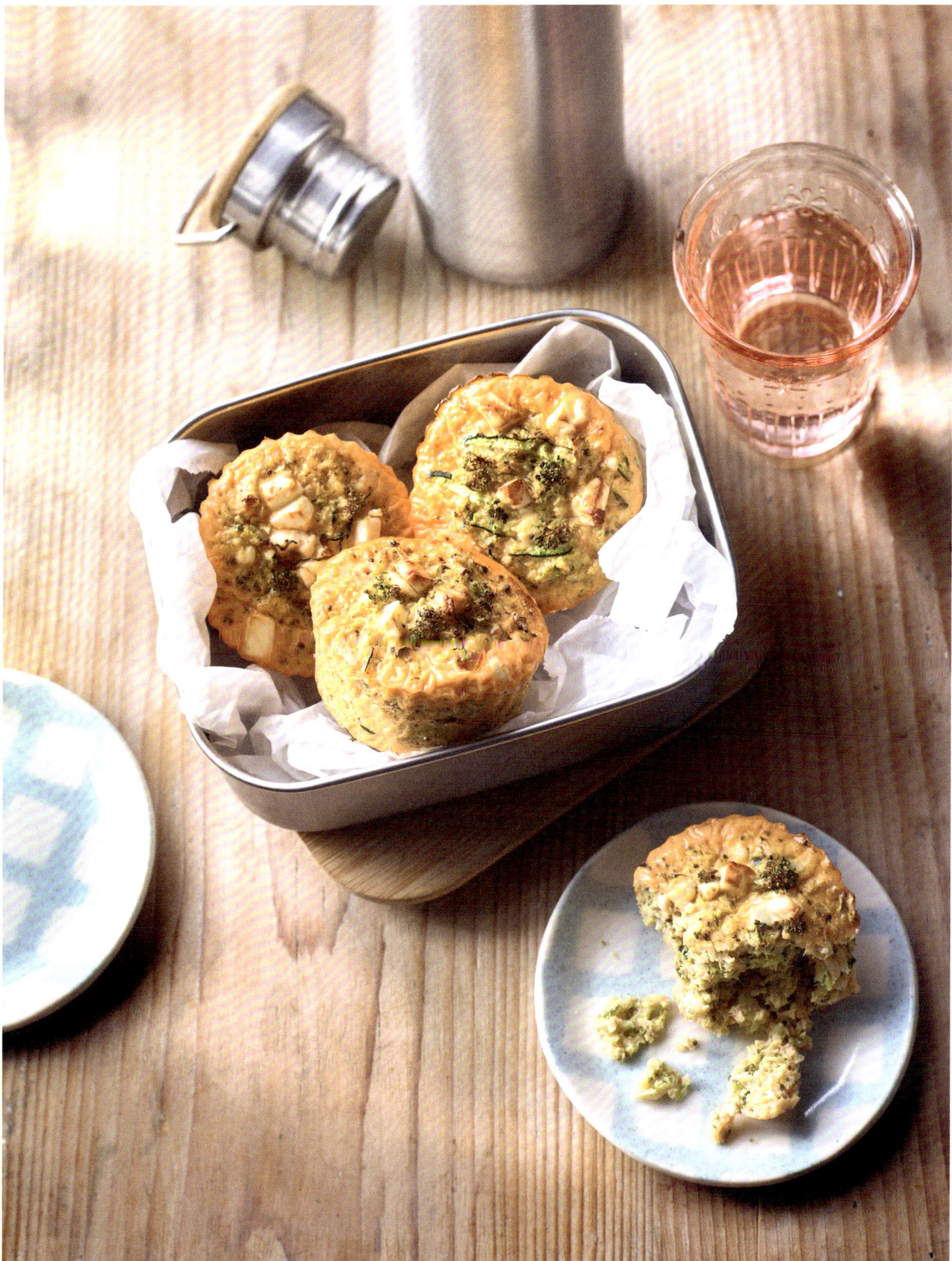

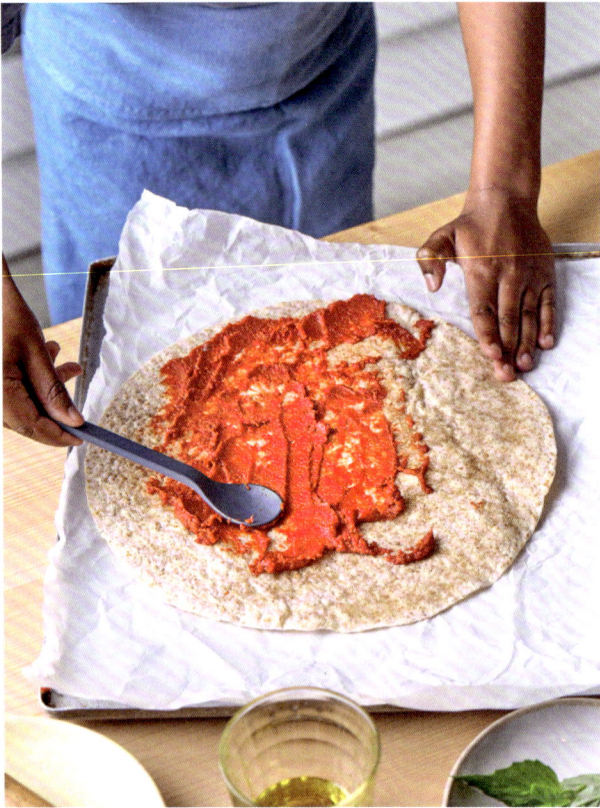

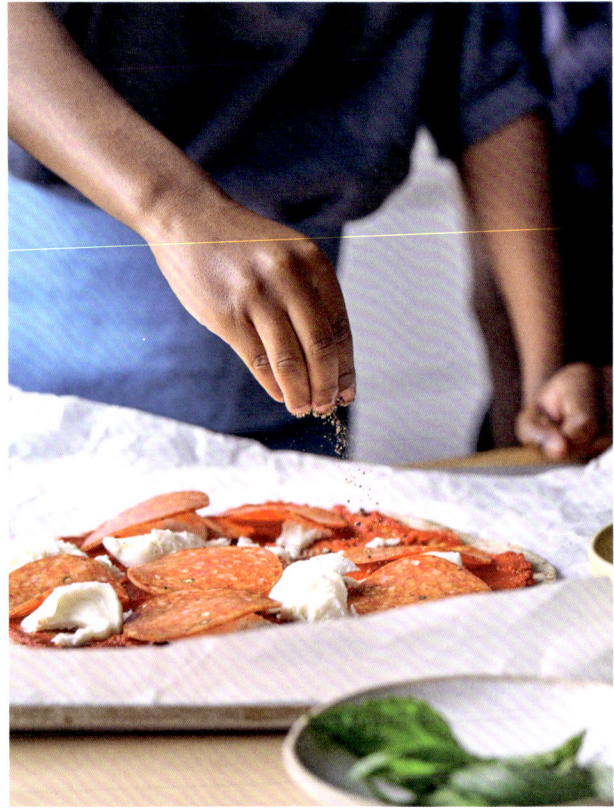

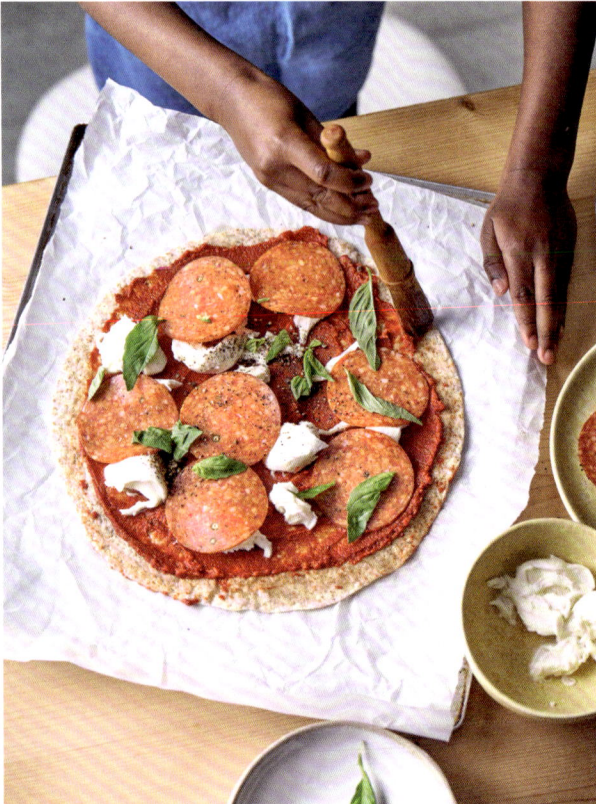

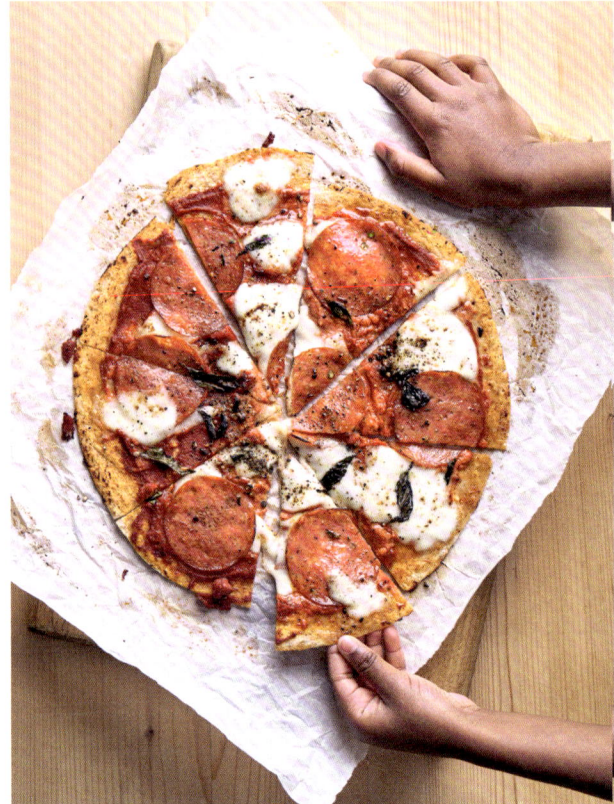

Easy Cheats Pizza

This cheats pizzas is a great way to rustle up a meal in no time at all that will delight all the family.

Prep time 5 minutes | **Cook time** 10 minutes | **Serves** 2

Ingredients
1 wholemeal tortilla wrap
1 tbsp tomato purée
1 ball of mozzarella, torn into pieces
6 slices of pepperoni or good-quality ham
A few fresh basil leaves (optional)
1 tsp olive oil

Method
1. Preheat the oven to 190°C/Fan 170°C/Gas 5 and line a large baking tray with non-stick baking paper.
2. Place the wrap on the prepared tray and spread the tomato purée all over. Scatter the mozzarella and pepperoni or ham over the wrap.
3. Brush the edges of the wrap with some of the olive oil. Season with salt and freshly ground black pepper and drizzle with the remaining olive oil.
4. Cook in the preheated oven for 10 minutes, or until the cheese is melted and golden, and the edges of the pizza are crisp.

Homemade Beans on Toast

These beans are almost identical in appearance to the tinned varieties, but are less processed and without the sugar. If you haven't had time to make the Six Veg Tomato Sauce, simply use the same quantity of tinned tomatoes in its place and season to taste.

Prep time 5 minutes | **Cook time** 20 minutes | **Serves** 2

Ingredients
1 × 400g tin haricot (or white) beans, drained and rinsed
350ml Six Veg Tomato Sauce (see page 164)
1 tbsp balsamic vinegar
4 slices of sourdough, toasted

Method
1. Place the beans, tomato sauce and vinegar in a saucepan over a medium heat. Simmer gently for 15–20 minutes, until the beans are soft and the sauce has reduced and thickened.
2. Spoon the beans on top of the toast to serve.

Sprinkling some grated Cheddar cheese over the top of these homemade beans makes a lovely addition.

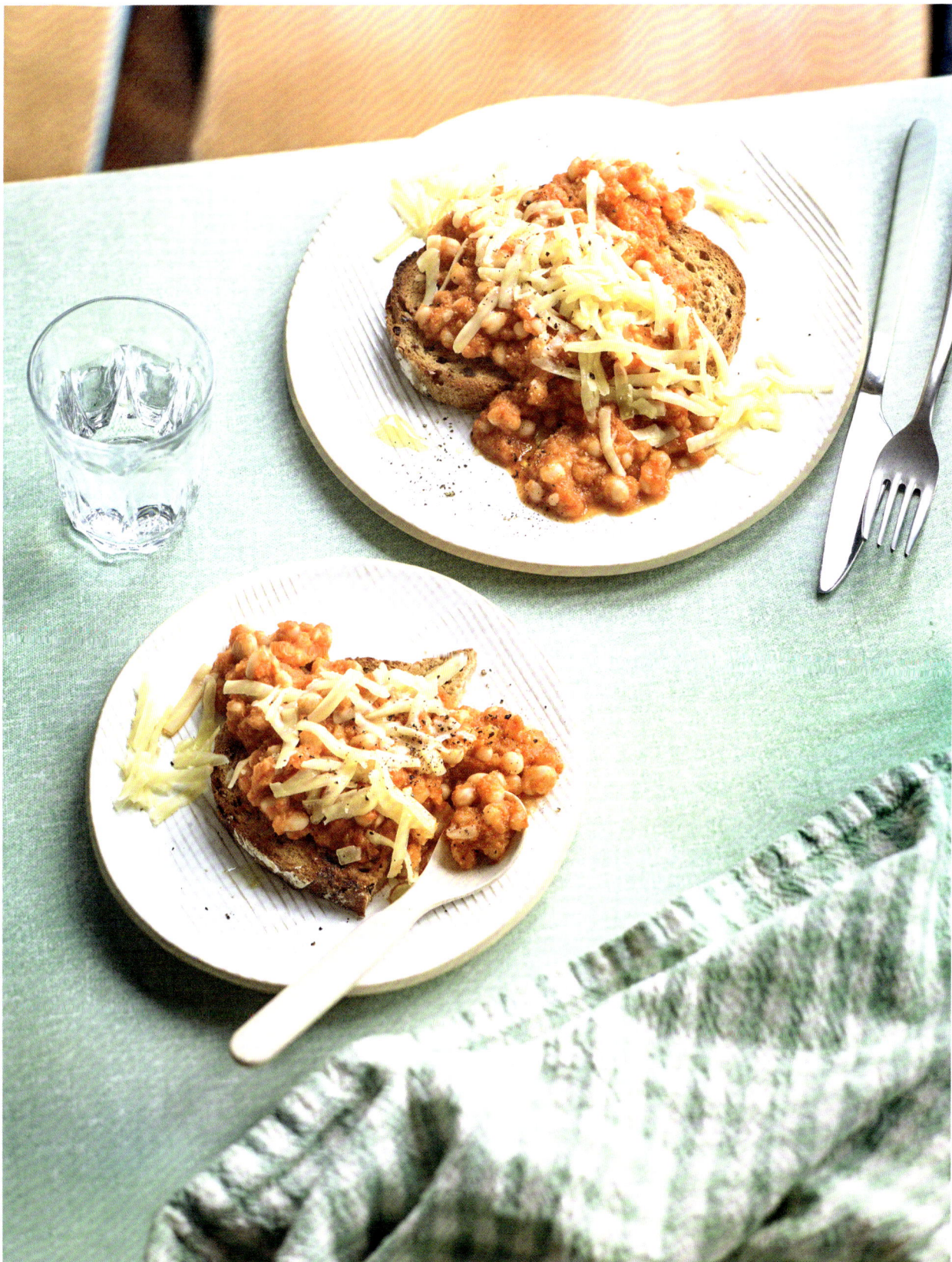

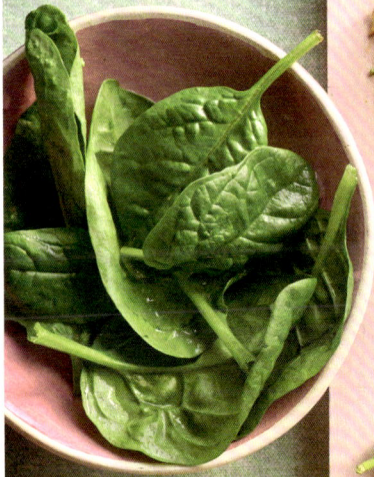

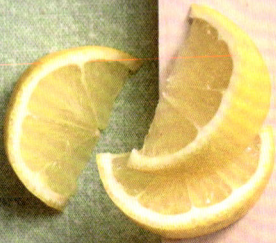

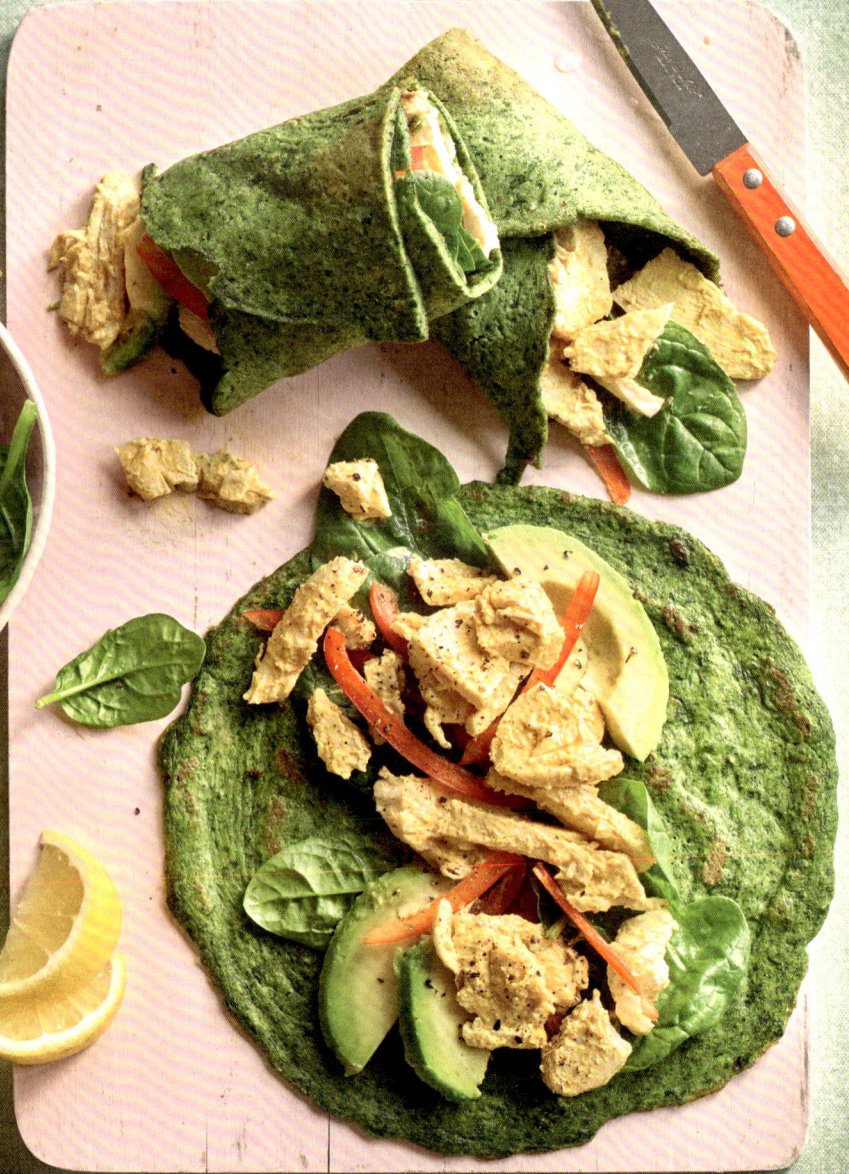

Spinach Wraps with Coronation Chicken

These are a fantastic alternative to shop-bought wraps and are full of protein. If using frozen spinach, defrost it first and squeeze out any excess water. These are delicious with the Parmesan-crusted Fish Nuggets (see page 120), for an elevated, delicious fish finger sandwich.

Prep time 20 minutes | **Cook time** 5 minutes | **Serves** 2–3

Ingredients

For the coronation chicken

300g cooked chicken, roughly chopped
1½ tsp mild curry powder
2 tbsp good-quality mayonnaise
2 tbsp full-fat Greek yoghurt
Juice of ¼ lemon

For the spinach wraps

2 medium eggs
1½ tbsp wholegrain flour
50g Cheddar, grated
50g fresh or frozen spinach, defrosted if frozen
1 tsp olive oil, for frying

Method

1. Mix all the coronation chicken ingredients together in a bowl and season with salt and freshly ground black pepper.
2. Place the spinach wrap ingredients in a jug or bowl and blitz using a stick blender until smooth – it should be a pourable consistency. Season with a little salt and pepper.
3. Swirl ½ teaspoon of olive oil around a large non-stick frying pan and place over a medium heat. Pour in half the batter and tilt the pan to spread it out evenly. Fry for 1 minute then carefully flip over. Fry for 1 minute on the other side, then transfer to a plate. Repeat with the remaining oil and batter and leave the wraps to cool.
4. When the wraps are cool, assemble with the coronation chicken and some salad ingredients, such as spinach leaves, sliced red pepper (capsicum) and avocado. Be careful with the delicate wraps when rolling.

Air Fryer Chicken Satay Skewers

These chicken skewers are a real favourite in recipe writer Kathryn's household and the children devour them as soon as they reach the table. Get ahead and make a double quantity of these, freeze them raw in batches and defrost them the morning you plan on cooking them. If you want to make these for a lunchbox, leave out the peanut butter – they'll still taste delicious.

Prep time 15 minutes | **Cook time** 12 minutes | **Serves** 4

Ingredients
1 tbsp olive oil
2cm piece of fresh ginger, finely grated
Juice of 1 lime
1 tsp honey or maple syrup
1½ tbsp soy sauce
1 tbsp mild curry powder
3 tbsp smooth peanut butter
2 chicken breasts, each sliced into 4 long, thin strips
8 × 18cm wooden skewers, soaked in water

Method
1. Place the olive oil, ginger, lime juice, honey or maple syrup, soy sauce, curry powder, peanut butter and a pinch of salt and some freshly ground pepper in a large bowl. Mix well until smooth, adding about 3 tablespoons of water to loosen the consistency. Add the chicken, toss to coat and leave to marinate for at least 30 minutes, or longer if possible.
2. Thread one strip of chicken onto each skewer, then place in the air fryer basket. Spoon over any excess marinade and cook at 200°C for 12 minutes, turning halfway through. Depending on the size of the air fryer, you may need to do this in batches.

In the absence of an air fryer, cook on a baking tray in an oven preheated to 200°C/Fan 180°C/Gas 6 for the same amount of time.

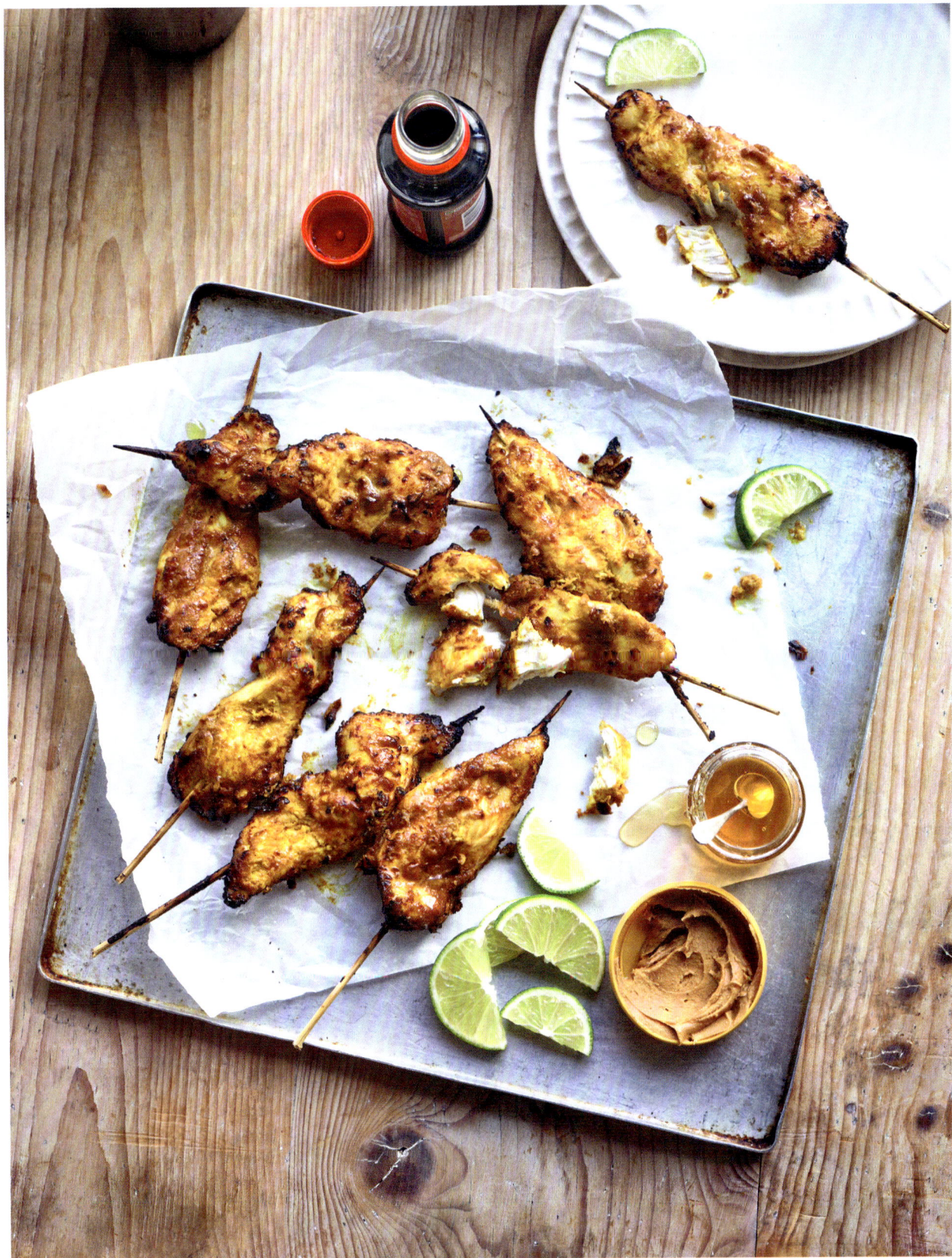

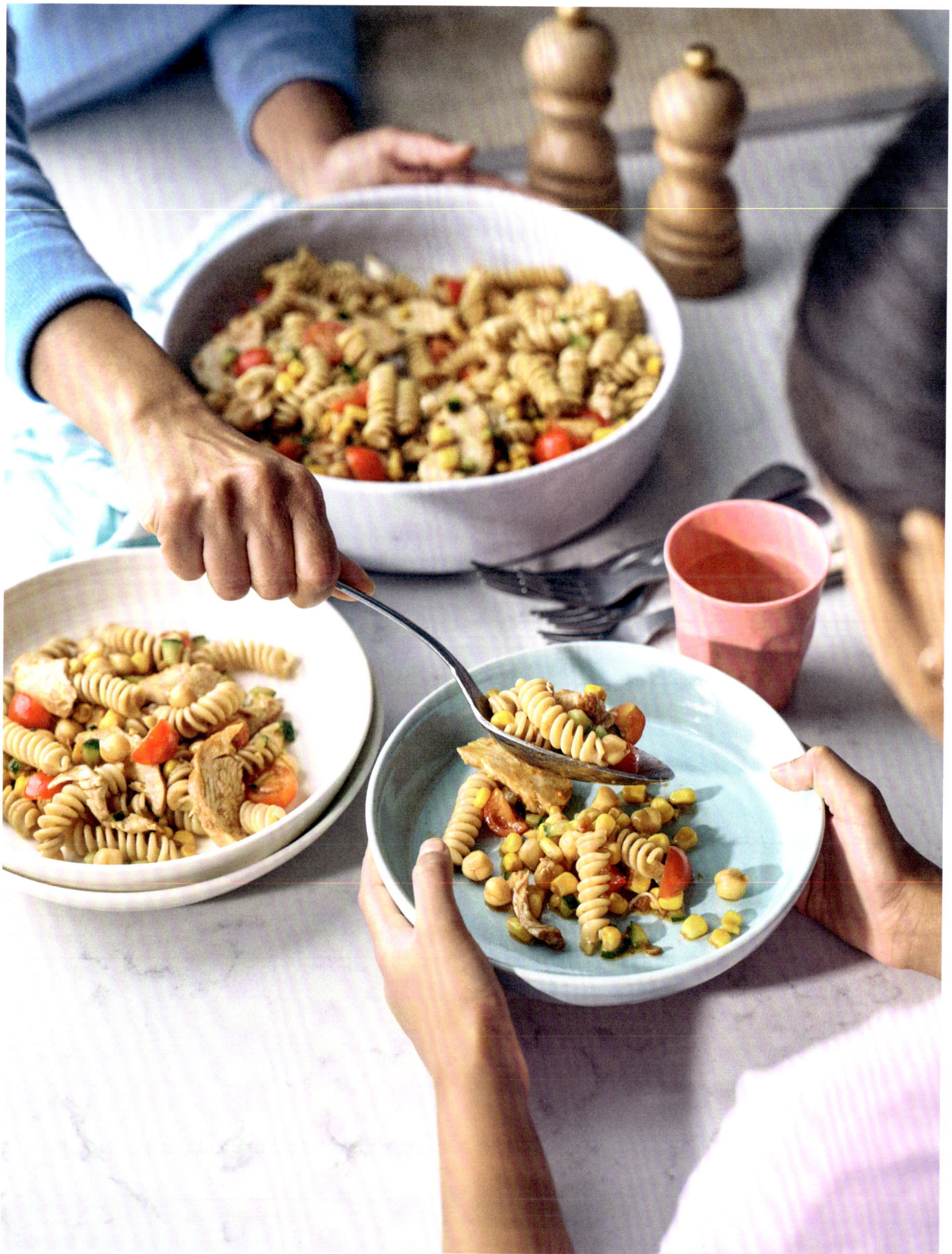

Traffic Light Protein Pasta Salad

This is a protein-rich pasta salad that lets you choose your main protein, along with sneaking in some fibre-rich pulses in the form of chickpeas. Go for one of the following to provide a bit more variety: 300g cooked chicken, finely diced, two 145g tins tuna, drained, or 300g Cheddar, cut into small cubes.

Prep time 10 minutes | **Cook time** 12 minutes | **Serves** 4

Ingredients
125g wholegrain fusilli pasta
½ x 400g tin chickpeas, drained and rinsed
12 cherry tomatoes, quartered (about 100g)
100g cucumber, finely diced
1 x 198g tin sweetcorn, drained
300g protein of choice (see intro)
1½ tbsp sun-dried tomato pesto
1 tsp balsamic vinegar

Method
1. Cook the pasta in a large pan of boiling salted water, according to packet instructions.
2. Drain the pasta and run under cold water to cool and stop the cooking. Transfer the pasta to a medium bowl.
3. Add all the remaining ingredients and toss to combine.
4. Season to taste with salt and freshly ground black pepper and serve.

Salmon Poke Bowl

This fabulous recipe came from a friend, Cecile Vadas, a young nutritionist in Sydney where poke bowls are elevated to a fine art. It is probably more suitable for older children. However, don't be deterred by the use of sriracha. Combined with yoghurt, it only gives a delicate heat and the overall combination of flavours and textures is truly delicious. You could use prawns instead of salmon, if preferred.

Prep time 15 minutes | **Cook time** 5 minutes | **Serves** 4

Ingredients
1 tsp honey
1 tsp finely grated fresh ginger
1 tsp sesame oil or olive oil, plus extra for frying
2 tsp soy sauce, plus extra to serve
4 salmon fillets
1 × 250g packet cooked wholegrain rice
80g frozen edamame beans, defrosted
1 avocado, peeled and finely diced
1 tbsp sesame seeds (optional)
3 tbsp full-fat Greek yoghurt
1 tbsp sriracha (optional)

Method
1. In a bowl, combine the honey, ginger, sesame or olive oil and soy sauce. Add the salmon and turn to coat. Leave to marinate for 30 minutes, if you have time.
2. Heat 1 teaspoon olive oil in a non-stick frying pan over a medium heat. Add the salmon and fry for 3–4 minutes, turning once, until just cooked.
3. Heat the rice according to the packet instructions and divide between four bowls, along with the edamame beans, avocado and sesame seeds, if using. Remove the skin from the cooked salmon fillets and flake the fish into the bowls.
4. Mix the yoghurt together with the sriracha, if using, and spoon over the fish. Serve with a little extra soy sauce on the side.

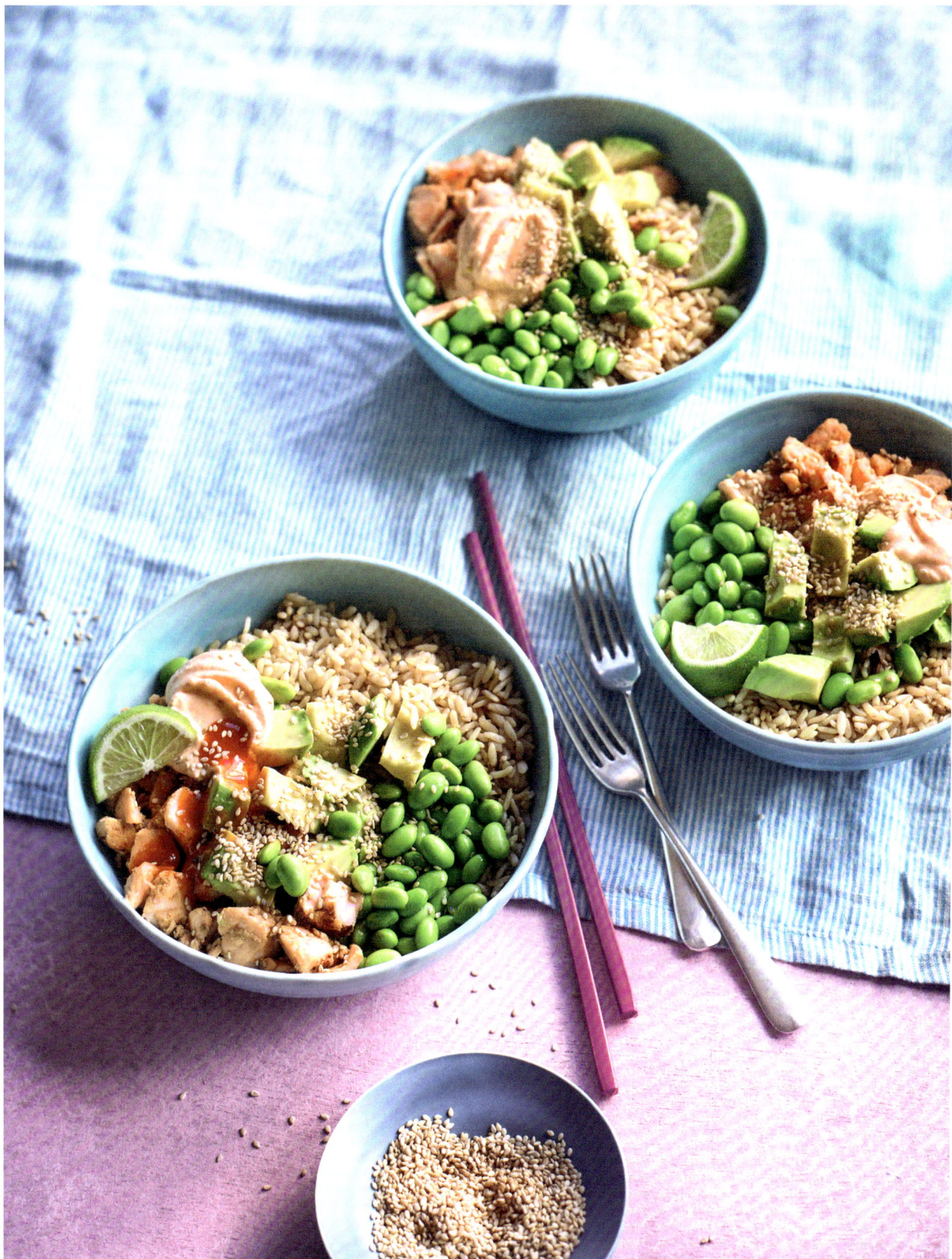

Snacks

Cheddar and Almond Biscuits

These are great little treats to sustain ravenous children! They are also great for crumbling on salads and soups for texture and added protein.

Prep time 15 minutes | **Cook time** 12 minutes | **Makes** 12

Ingredients
200g Cheddar, grated
100g ground almonds
1 tbsp ground flaxseed (or whole golden flaxseed)
1 medium or large egg white, lightly whisked

Method
1. Preheat the oven to 180°C/Fan 160°C/Gas 4. Line a large baking tray with non-stick baking paper.
2. Mix all the ingredients except the egg white in a medium bowl.
3. Add the egg white and 1 tablespoon of water. Using a wooden spoon, mix vigorously to form a crumbly dough.
4. Scoop a tablespoon at a time of the mixture into your hands and roll tightly into the shape of a golf ball. The mixture should make 12 biscuits.
5. Place the balls on the prepared baking tray, spaced apart, and use the back of a fork to flatten to 1cm thickness. Bake in the preheated oven for 10–12 minutes, until golden brown and crisping.
6. Transfer carefully to a wire rack and leave to cool, where they will crisp up further.

Add a pinch of chilli flakes to the mixture to turn these into a delicious adult snack.

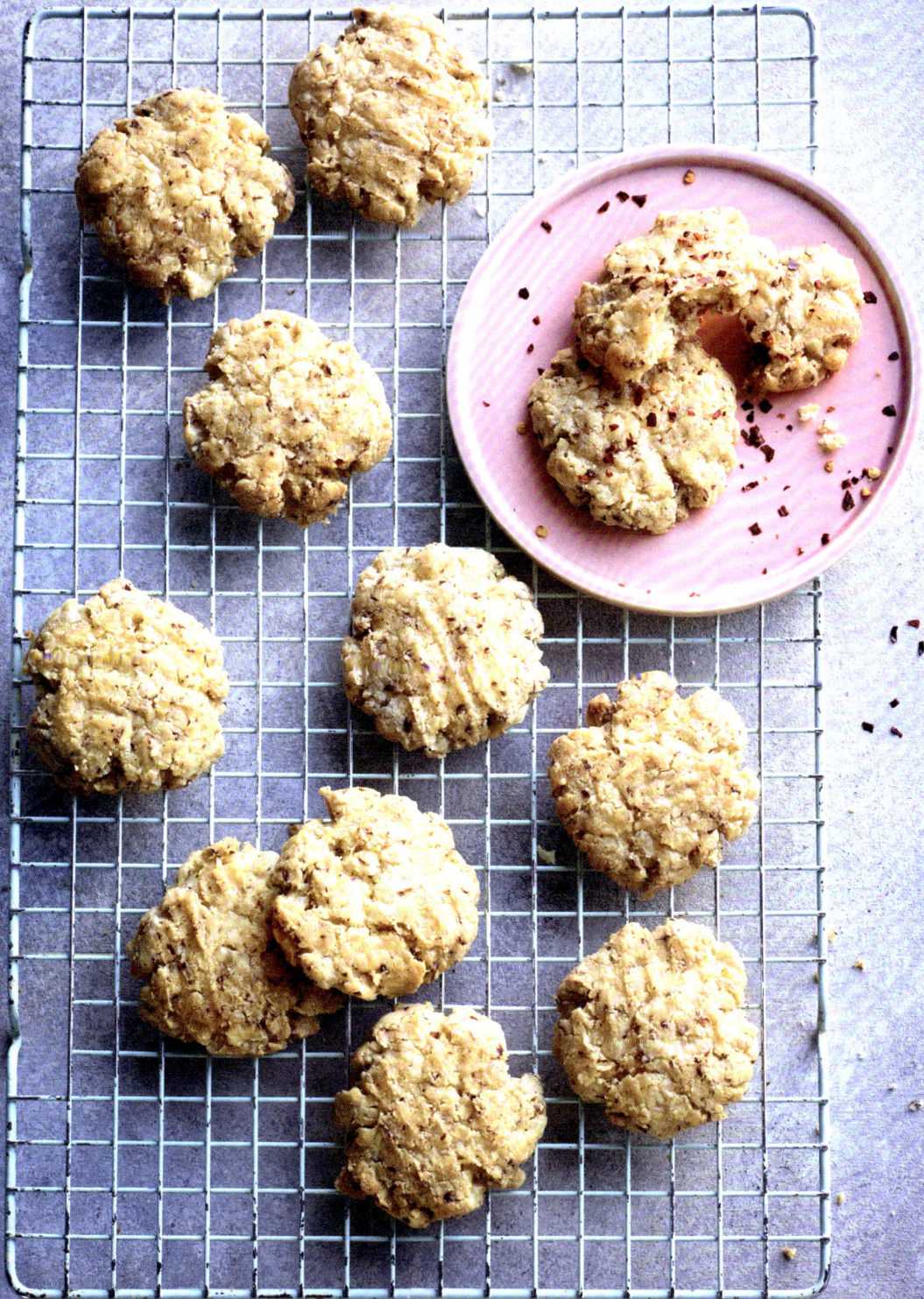

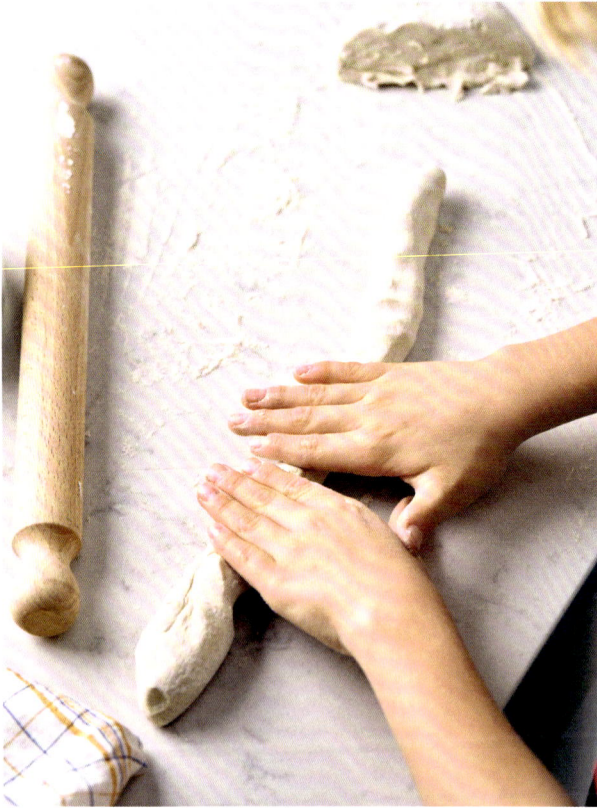

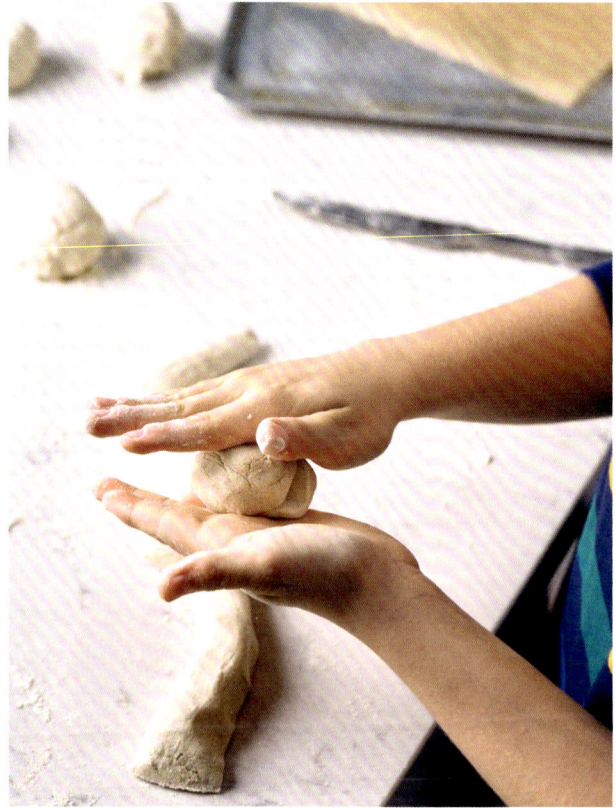

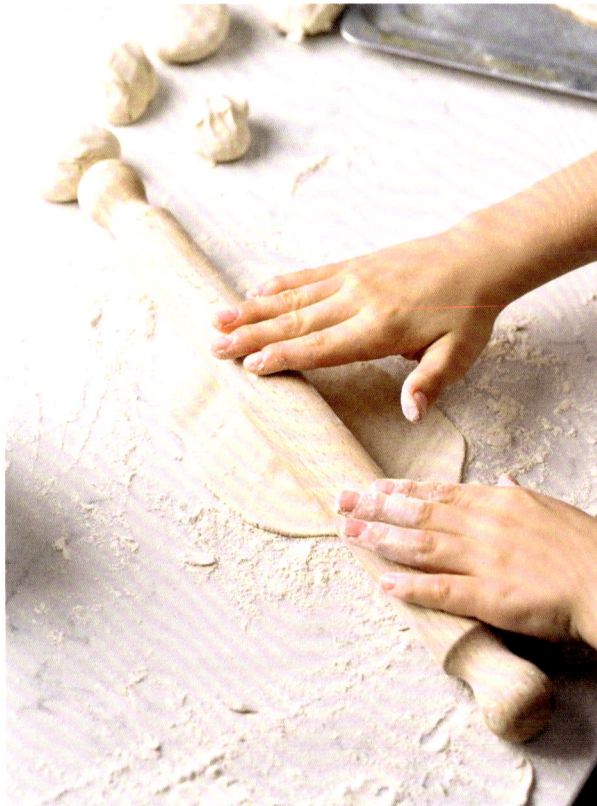

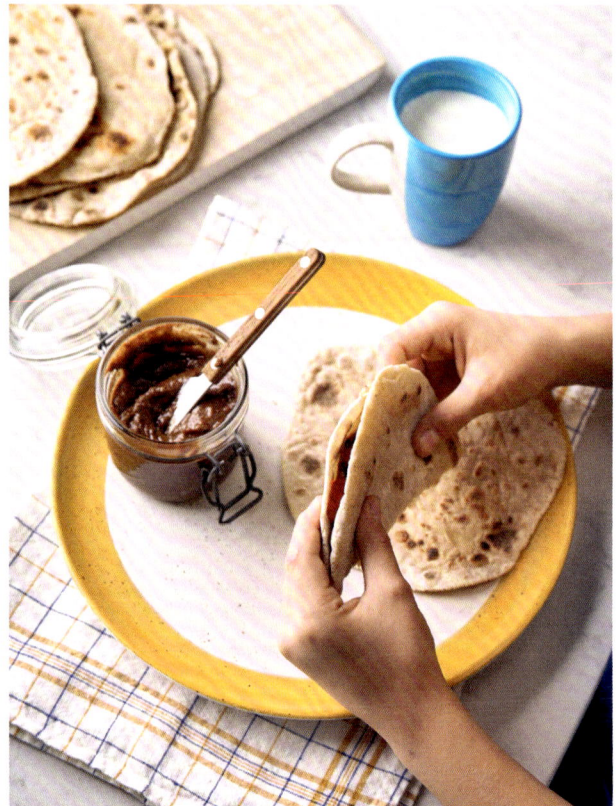

Gluten-free Buckwheat Wraps

These delicious wraps are perfect for lunch boxes. Brush them with a little olive oil and serve them with dips, use a wrap instead of bread for a sandwich, or serve them alongside stews to mop up delicious sauces. They are also lovely with Crunchy Homemade Chocolate Spread (see page 173).

Prep time 15 minutes | **Cook time** 30 minutes | **Makes** 8

Ingredients
175g buckwheat flour, plus extra for dusting
230g full-fat Greek yoghurt
Olive oil, to finish

Method
1. Place the flour and yoghurt in a large bowl with a generous pinch of salt. Use a wooden spoon to mix until the mixture begins to form a dough.
2. Tip out onto a lightly floured surface and knead gently to form a smooth ball. Roll the dough into a long log and cut into eight equal pieces. Dust the work surface with a bit more flour, if necessary, and roll each piece to a thin disc about 13cm diameter.
3. Place a large frying pan over a high heat and, when hot, add a wrap and cook for 2 minutes on each side, until puffed and golden brown. As each one is ready, brush with some olive oil and season with a generous pinch of salt.
4. Serve immediately. Otherwise, store the wraps in the fridge for up to 2 days. Reheat them in the microwave, as needed.

Seeded Parmesan Crackers

It is hard to find healthy and substantial snacks to feed hungry mouths. These biscuits will be a big hit – cheesy, crispy and delicious. They are easy to prepare and can be made in moments. If you have some Parmesan in the fridge and a pack of mixed seeds in your cupboard, you are moments away from a nutritious and tasty snack for the family.

Prep time 10 minutes | **Cook time** 8 minutes | **Makes** 12

Ingredients
150g Parmesan, finely grated
2–3 tbsp mixed seeds

Method
1. Preheat the oven to 180°C/Fan 160°C/Gas 4 and line two baking trays with non-stick baking paper.
2. Mix the grated Parmesan with the seeds in a bowl.
3. Use a tablespoon to make small piles on the prepared baking trays, leaving a little space between each one. Press down to make uniform discs, roughly the size of cookies. Bake in the preheated oven for about 8 minutes, until golden and crisp.
4. Leave to cool completely on the tray before transferring to a plate or wire rack.

The crackers will keep for a couple of days in an airtight container.

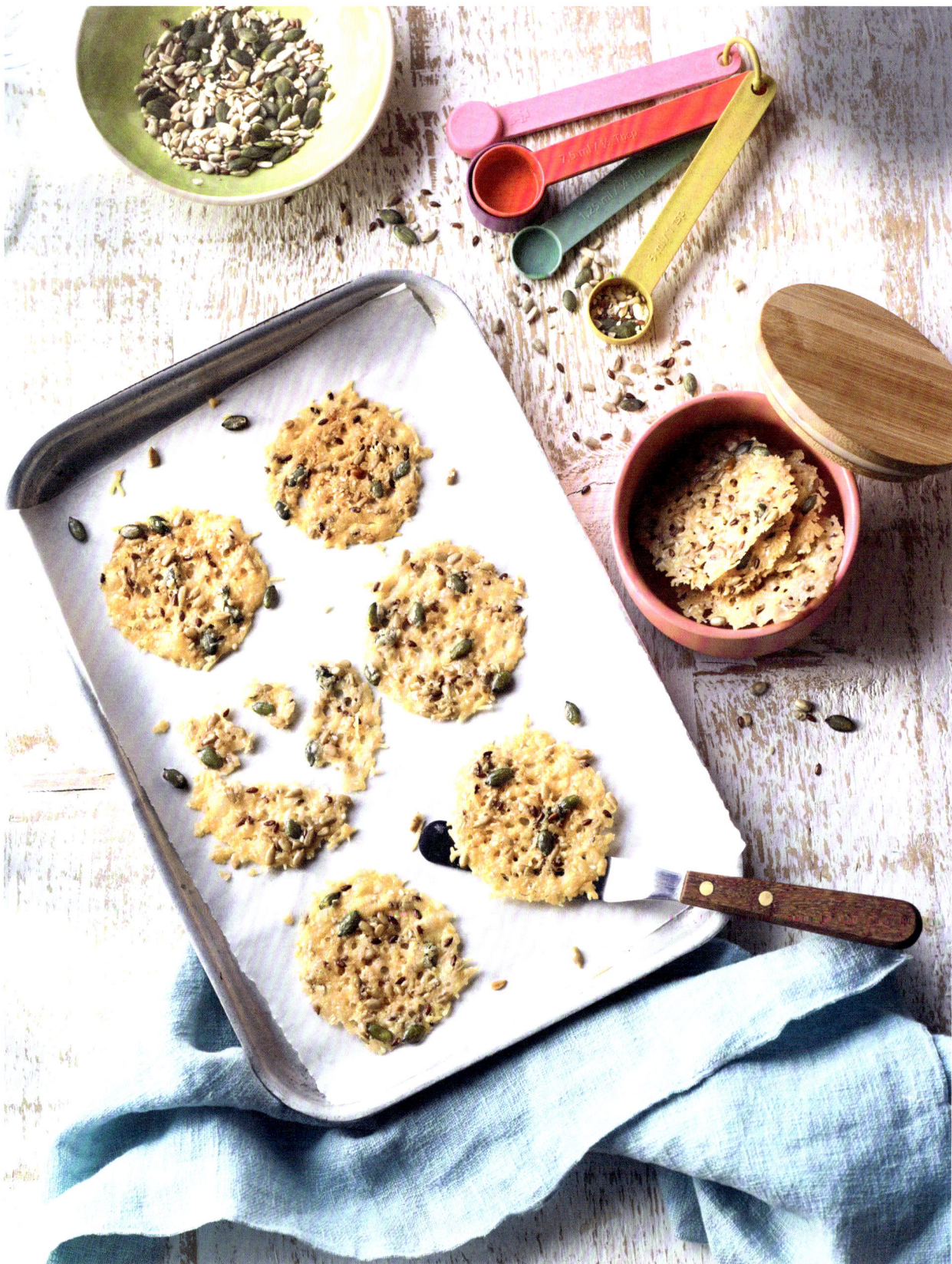

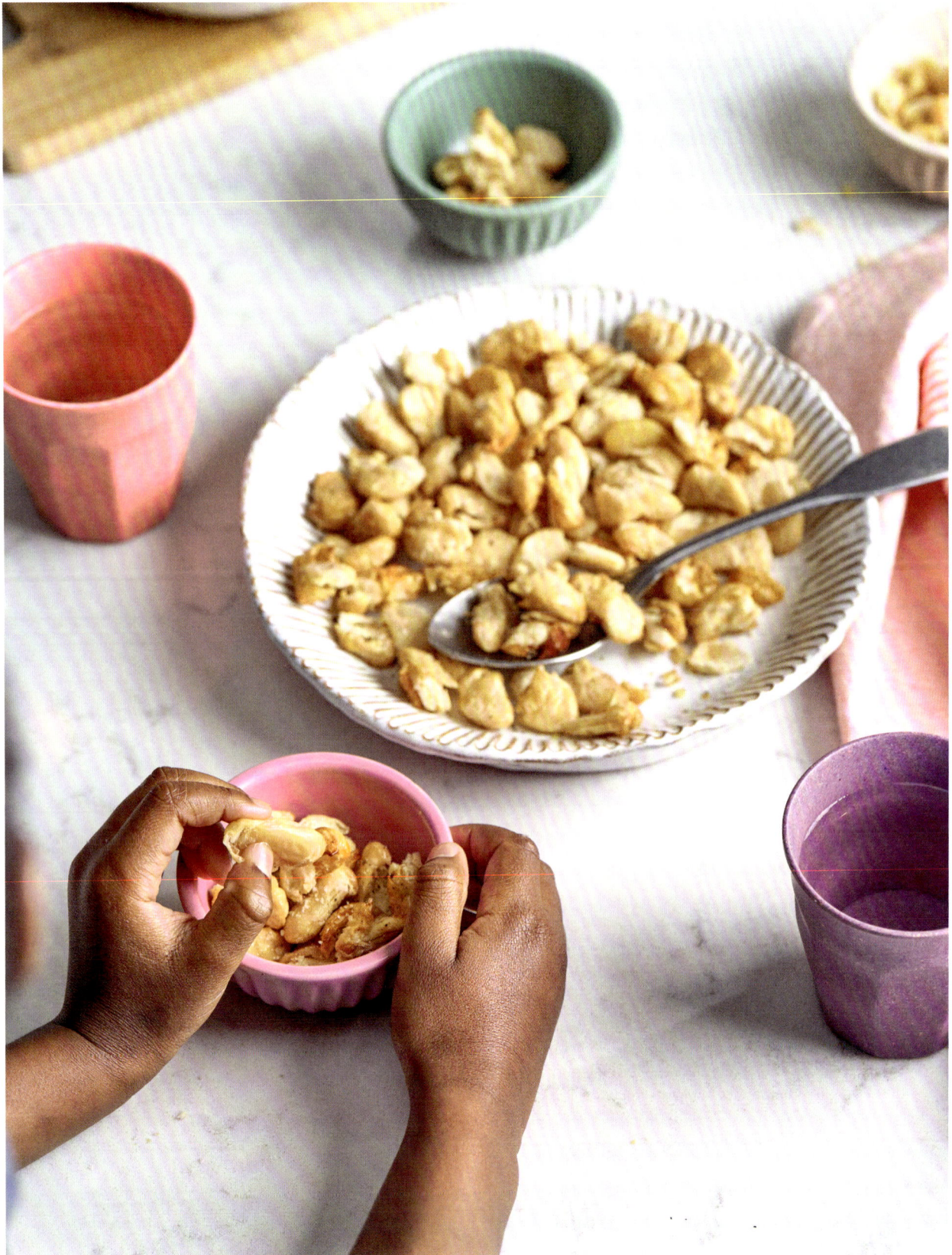

Air Fryer Garlic Butter Beans

Butter beans can make a great crispy little snack, and are a good substitute for chips. Probably not suited for young children, due to possible choking.

Prep time 5 minutes | **Cook time** 8 minutes | **Serves** 4

Ingredients
1 × 400g tin butter beans, drained and rinsed
2 tbsp olive oil
1 garlic clove, finely grated

Method
1. Place the butter beans on some kitchen paper and pat dry. Transfer to a bowl with 1½ tablespoons of the olive oil, the garlic and a pinch of salt and freshly ground black pepper. Toss to coat.
2. Cook in the air fryer at 200°C for 8 minutes, until golden and bursting open.
3. Dress with the remaining olive oil to serve.

These beans will also cook well for 8 minutes in an oven preheated to 220°C/Fan 200°C/Gas 7. Simply tip onto a baking tray lined with non-stick baking paper and toss halfway through the cooking time.

Beetroot Falafels

Most kids like food that is presented in bite-sized nuggets, as are these falafels. These lovely, crunchy balls are also marvellously purple, so they will do well on the 'eat a rainbow' challenge.

Prep time 10 minutes | **Cook time** 25 minutes | **Makes** 12

Ingredients
1 × 400g tin chickpeas, drained and rinsed
2 vacuum-packed cooked beetroot (about 100g)
70g feta, crumbled
Zest of 1 lemon
1½ tbsp wholemeal spelt flour (or other wholemeal flour)

Method
1. Preheat the oven to 200°C/Fan 180°C/Gas 6 and line a baking tray with non-stick baking paper.
2. Place all the ingredients in a large bowl with a pinch of salt and some freshly ground black pepper. Blend with a stick blender until almost smooth. (It is nice to leave some whole chickpeas for texture.)
3. Shape into 12 golf-ball-sized falafels (damp hands will help with this) and place on the prepared baking tray. Bake in the preheated oven for 25 minutes, until firm.
4. Leave to cool before serving.

These falafels are delicious served with Cucumber in Yoghurt (see page 168).

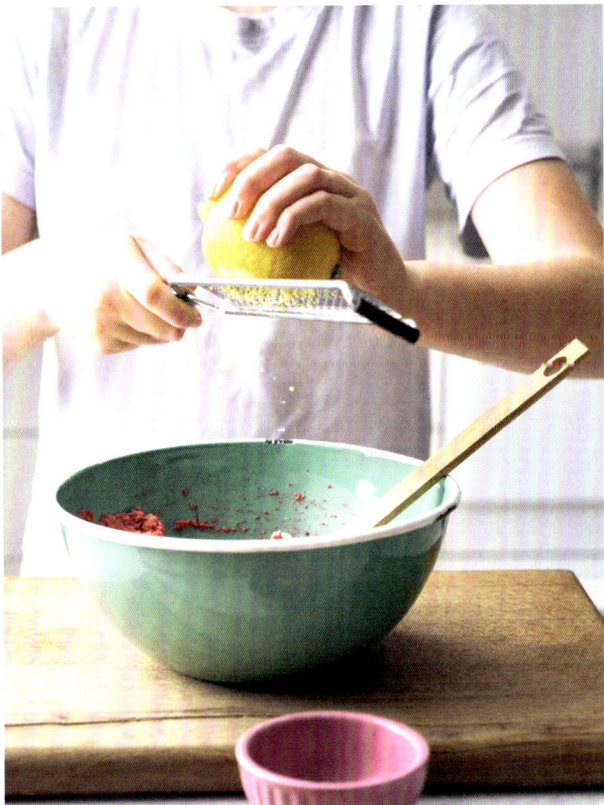

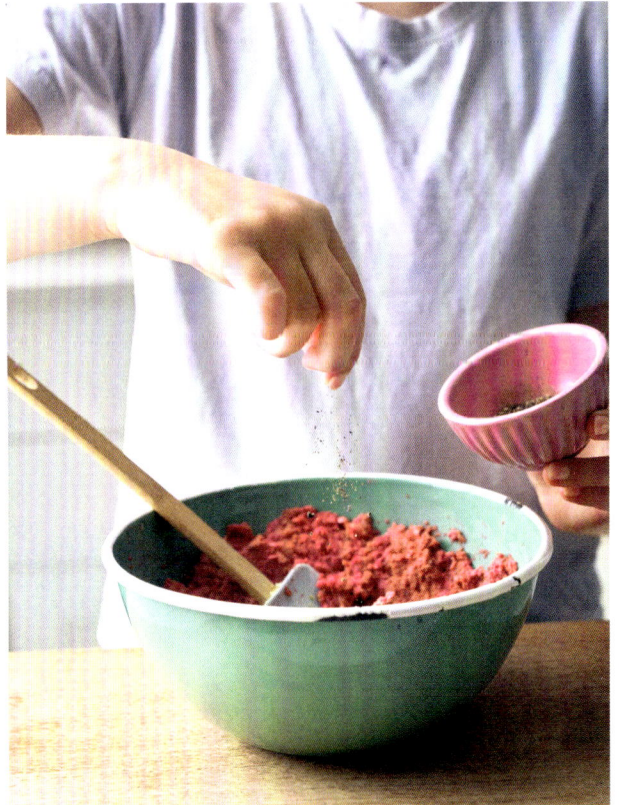

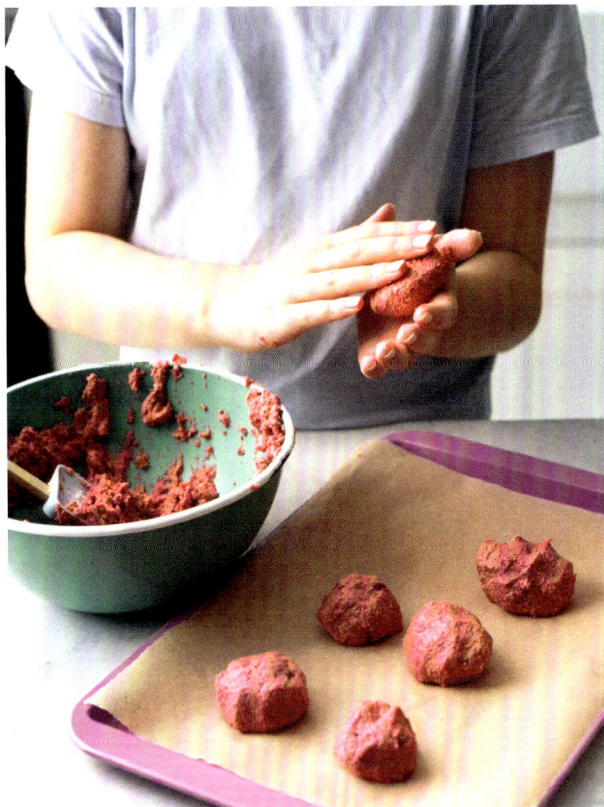

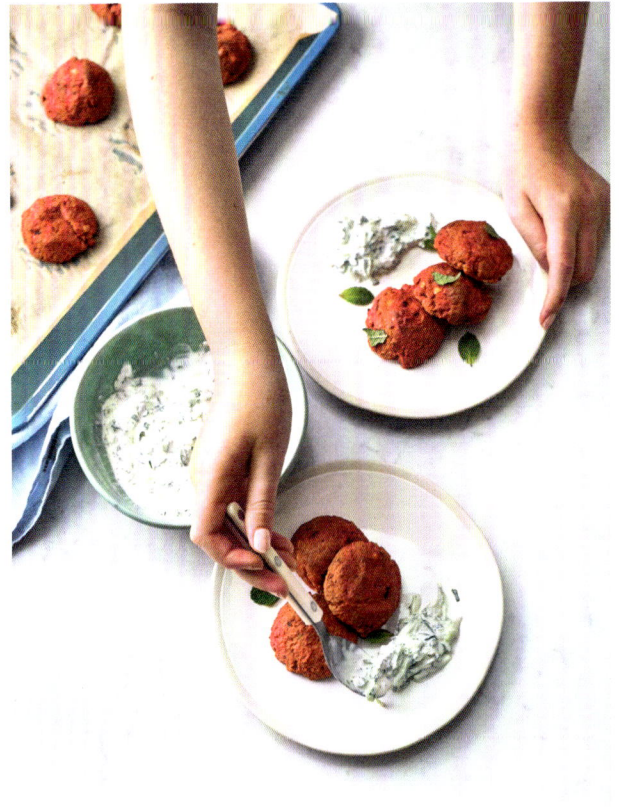

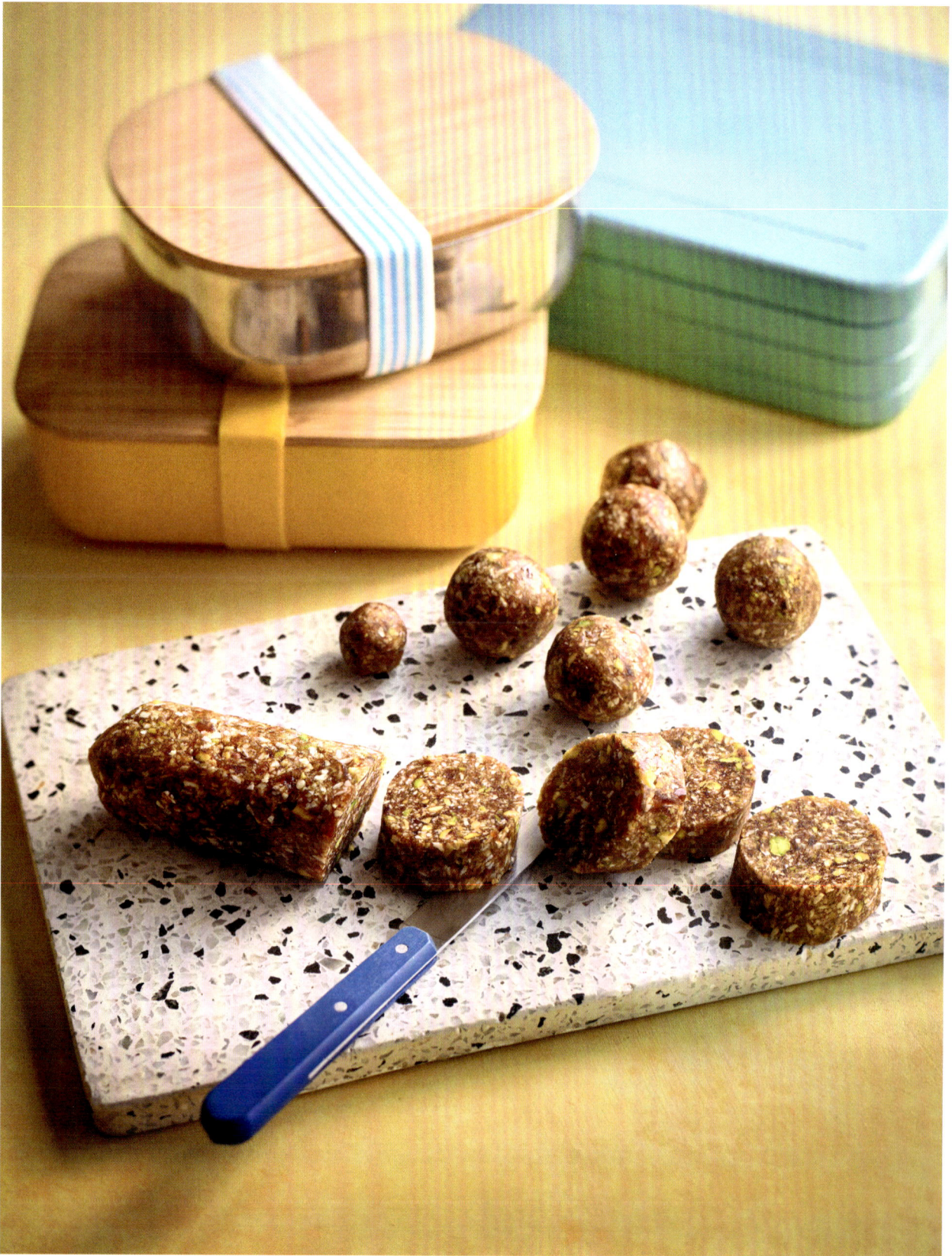

Protein Power Balls

These highly nutritious power balls are a favourite of our grown-up children. Packed with fibre, protein and omega-3, they are so easy to make. Slightly sweet and delicately flavoured, these treats are mildly nutty and totally irresistible.

Prep time 8 minutes | Makes 10

Ingredients
2 tbsp chopped pistachios (or nuts of choice)
2 tbsp desiccated coconut
2 tbsp ground almonds
9 soft pitted dates, diced
½ tsp ground cinnamon

Method
1. Place all the ingredients in a food processor and blitz for 1–2 minutes, leaving some texture. (Alternatively, you can do this with a stick blender.)
2. Shape the mixture into a thin log, then cut into 10 equal pieces. Roll each piece into a ball.
3. Enjoy straight away or place in a sealed container and store in the fridge.

The balls will keep in the fridge for up to 2 weeks.

Chocolate Popcorn

This delicious popcorn is a treat that won't cause a sugar frenzy! Note that it is not suitable for young children, due to the risk of choking.

Prep time 5 minutes | **Cook time** 2 minutes | **Serves** 6

Ingredients
1 tsp olive oil
2 tbsp popcorn kernels (about 30g)
60g dark chocolate (at least 70% cocoa solids), melted

Method
1. Place the olive oil and popcorn kernels in a medium saucepan with a tight-fitting lid. Place the pan over a high heat and pop the corn for 1–2 minutes. When the popping slows down, turn off the heat and leave for a few seconds longer until the popping stops altogether.
2. Tip the popcorn out onto a large baking tray in a single layer to cool.
3. Drizzle the melted chocolate all over the cooled popcorn, then sprinkle with a pinch of sea salt. Transfer to the fridge to set.
4. Break into chunks to serve.

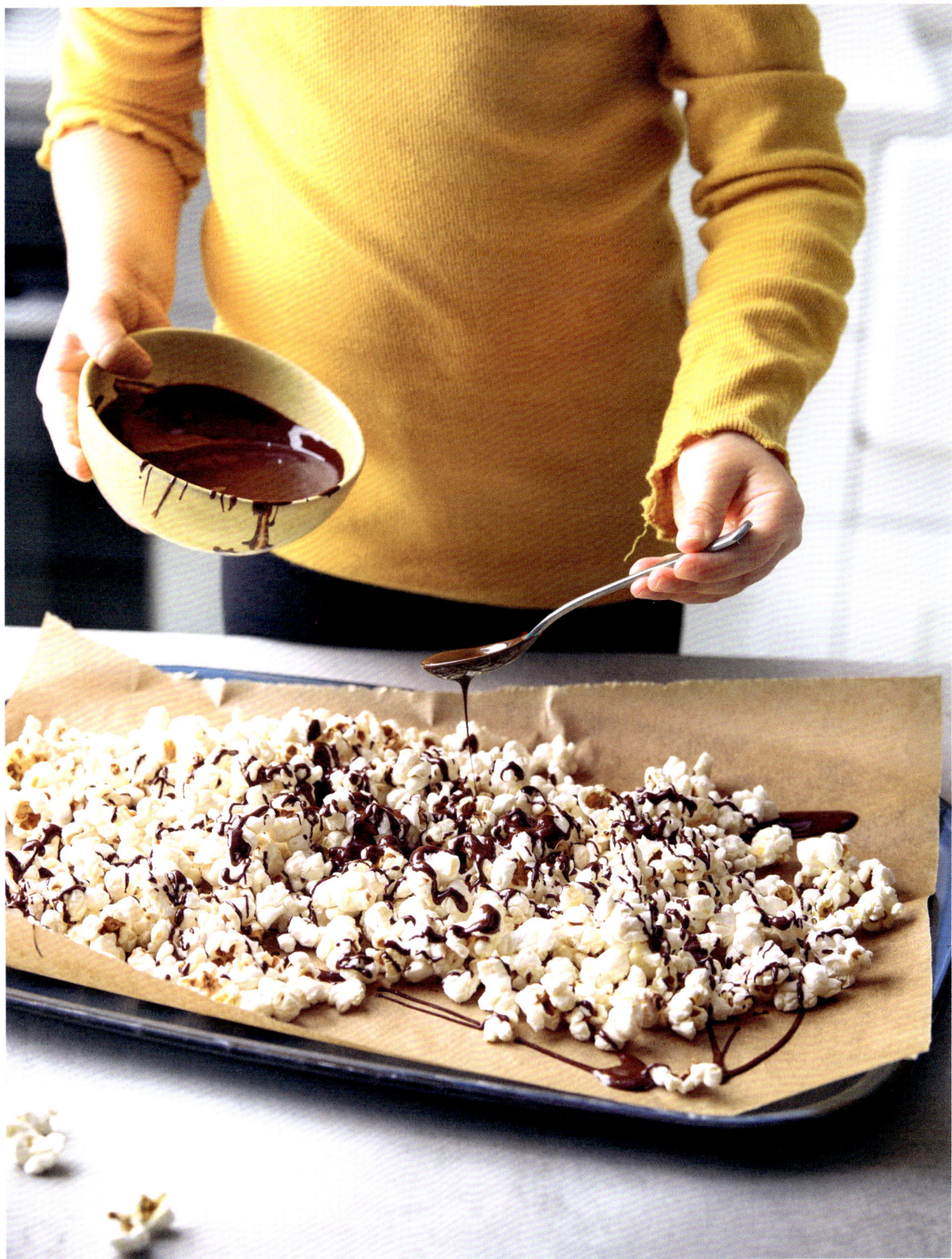

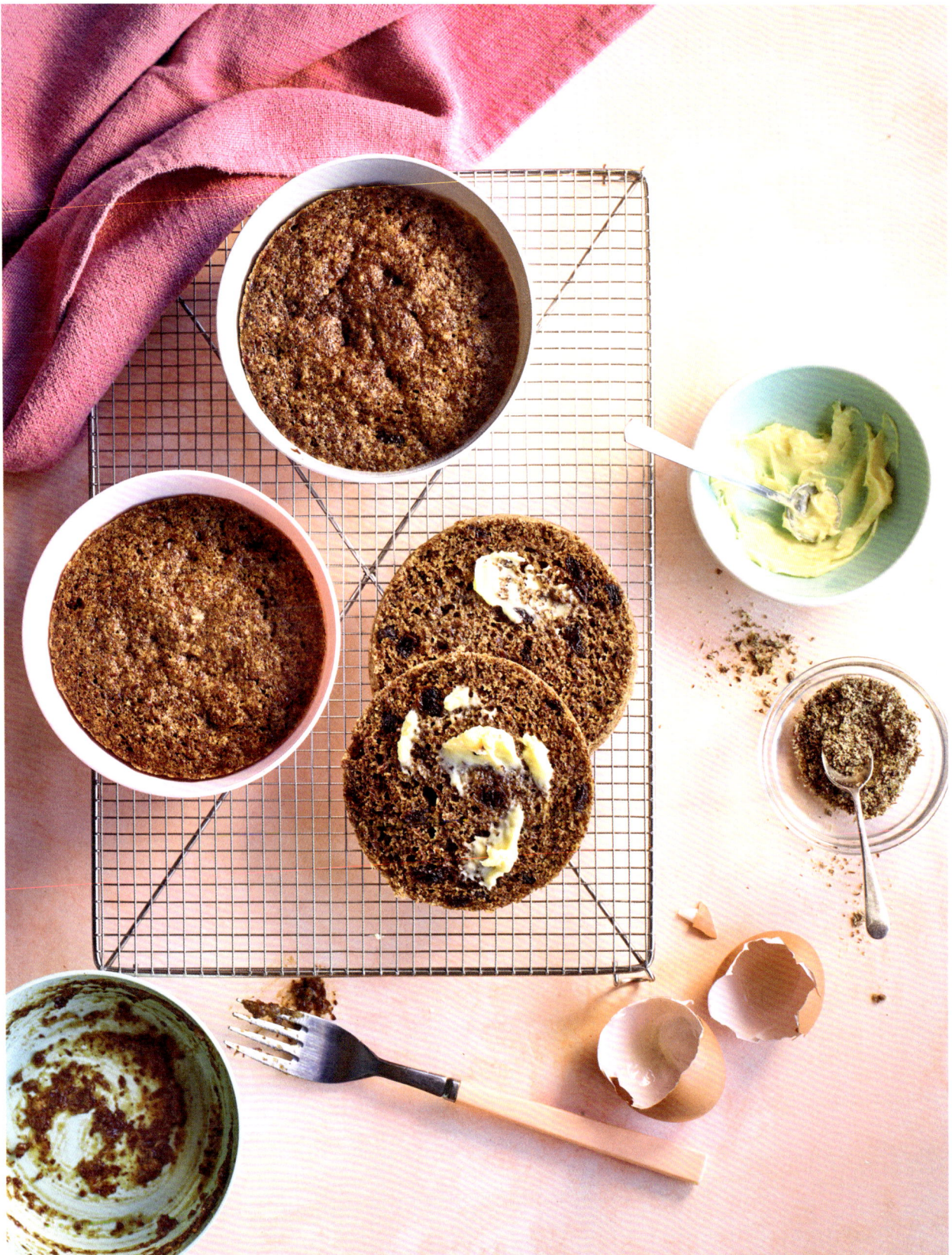

Mixed Spice Instant Muffin

We do enjoy an instant muffin! This is a bit like a fruit bun with a comforting spiced flavour. It's also rich in protein, too. This is delicious sliced in half and toasted with butter.

Prep time 5 minutes | **Cook time** 70 seconds | **Serves** 2

Ingredients
½ tbsp coconut oil, melted
4 tbsp ground flaxseed
1 medium egg
½ tsp baking powder
½ tsp mixed spice
1 tbsp maple syrup
1 tbsp sultanas

Method
1. Measure the ingredients into a heatproof bowl or large heatproof mug (about 8–10cm diameter). Make sure it is big enough for the mixture to rise as it cooks. Add a pinch of salt and mix until smooth.
2. Microwave on high for 1 minute. If the surface is still soft, return to the microwave for another 10 seconds, or until firm.
3. Tip out onto a clean surface and leave to cool.

Spelt Soda Bread

This bread is remarkably easy to make – no weighing scales required, just a mug from the kitchen cupboard. If you add ground flaxseed for extra fibre, you may need an extra splash of water in the dough. You can bake this in a loaf tin for easy slicing, or form it into a traditional round and cook on a baking tray.

Prep time 10 minutes | **Cook time** 50 minutes | **Makes** 1 loaf

Ingredients
2 mugs white spelt flour
1 mug rolled or jumbo oats
½ mug ground flaxseed (optional)
1 tsp bicarbonate of soda
1 tsp sea salt
¾ mug full-fat Greek yoghurt
2 tbsp honey

Method
1. Preheat the oven to 180°C/Fan 160°C/Gas 4 and line a loaf tin or baking tray with non-stick baking paper.
2. Use a mug to measure the flour, oats and ground flaxseed, if using, into a bowl. Add the bicarbonate of soda and salt, and mix well to combine.
3. Add the yoghurt and honey to the dry ingredients and mix thoroughly until you have a slightly sticky dough – add a splash of water, if needed.
4. Tip the dough into the prepared loaf tin, if using, pressing down to level the top. Otherwise, shape the dough into a rough ball and place on the prepared baking tray. Cut a 1cm-deep cross into the dough and sprinkle with a few extra oats. Bake in the preheated oven for 50 minutes.
5. Transfer to a wire rack to cool before slicing.

This bread freezes brilliantly. It is easier to slice this loaf before it goes in the freezer. I often keep sliced bread in the freezer and stick it straight in the toaster. There is evidence that by freezing and defrosting starchy foods like bread, some of the fibres change to what is called resistant starch, which your gut microbiome loves. Keep those lovely bugs healthy and they will do the same for you!

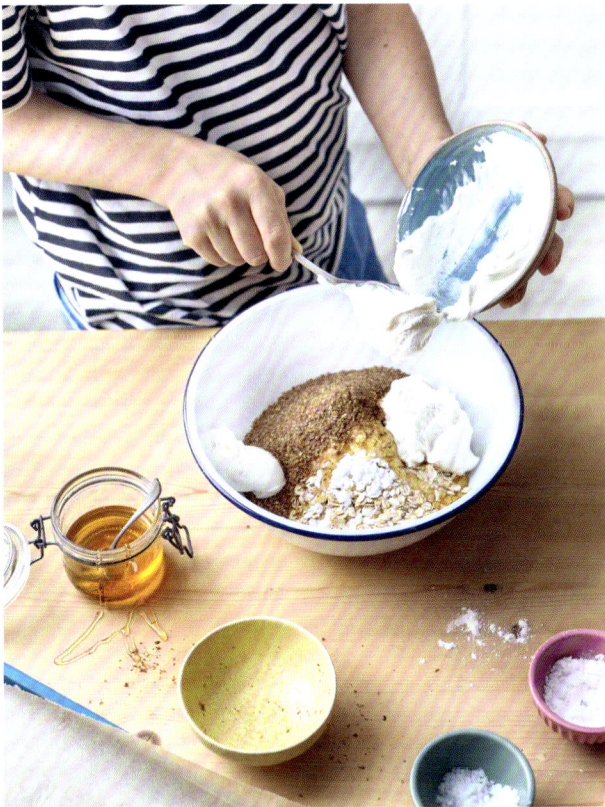
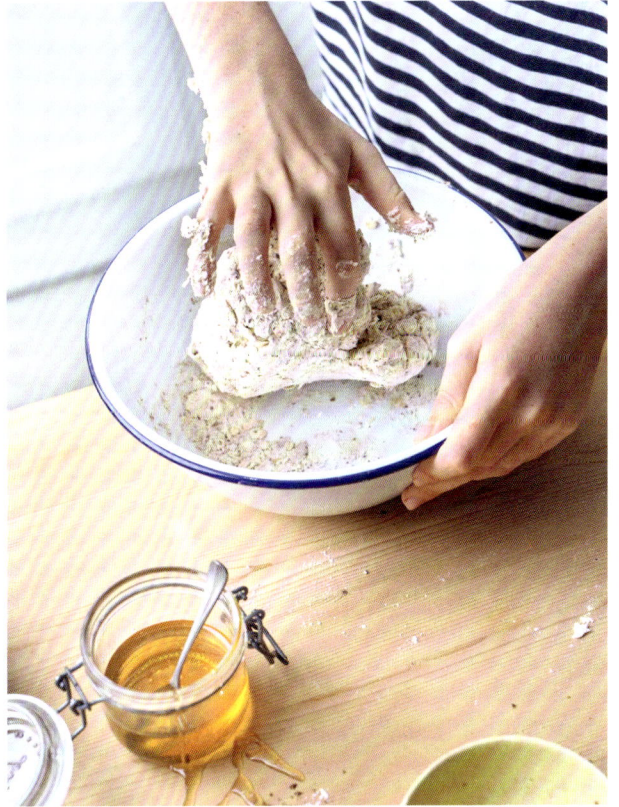
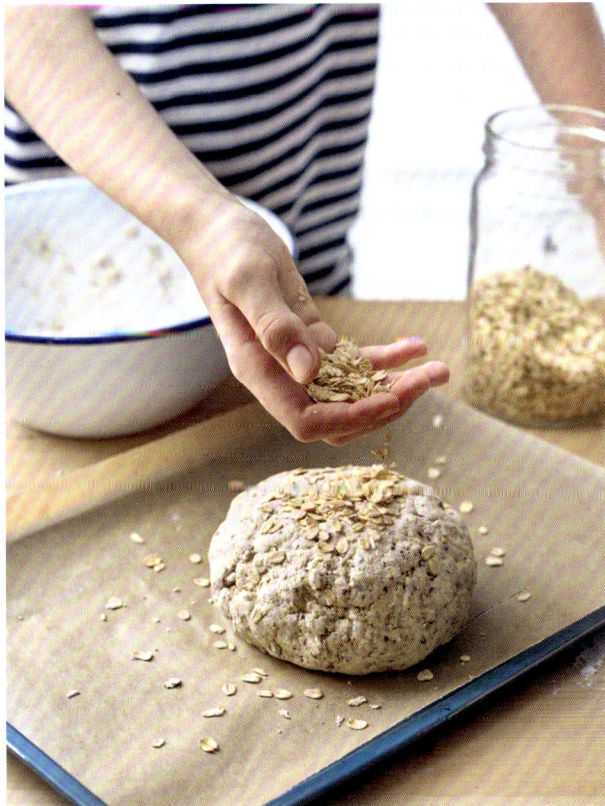
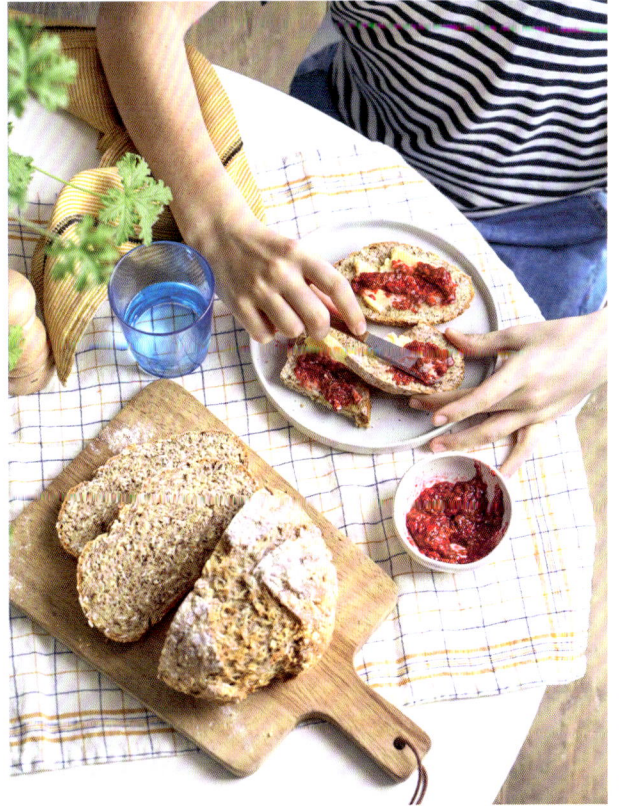

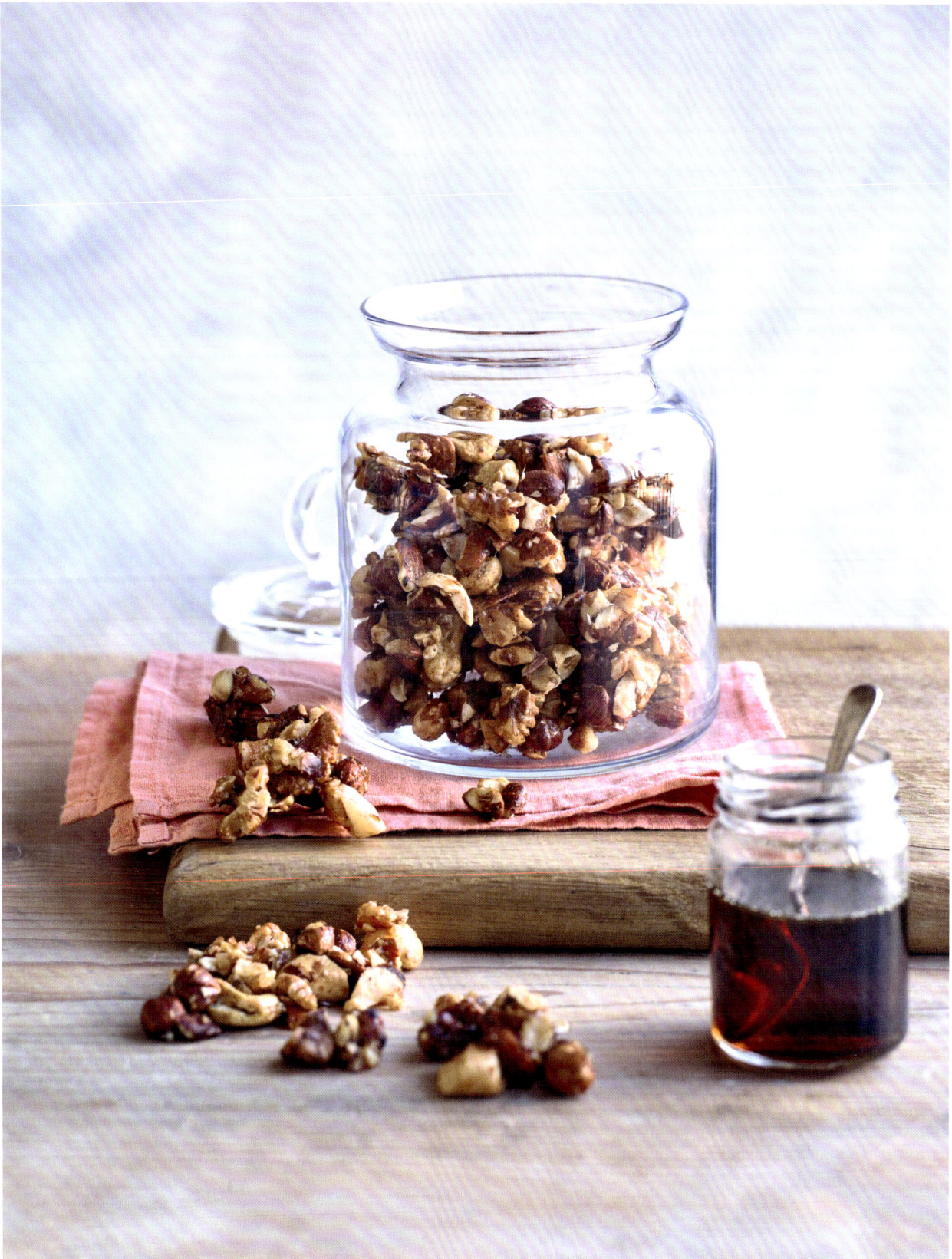

Sticky Nut Clusters

Getting little ones into the habit of eating nuts is fantastic if you can achieve it. These clusters will help to introduce nuts as an everyday snack. They are deliciously crispy, and a little sweet and aromatic with cinnamon. Buy a bag of mixed nuts and make a batch of these clusters at the beginning of the week, and offer them as an alternative to ultra-processed snacks. These clusters are not appropriate for very small children.

Prep time 5 minutes | **Cook time** 7 minutes | **Makes** 8

Ingredients
225g mixed nuts, roughly chopped
3 tbsp maple syrup
1 tsp ground cinnamon

Method
1. Preheat the oven to 180°C/Fan 160°C/Gas 4 and line a baking tray with non-stick baking paper.
2. In a medium bowl, combine the nuts, maple syrup, cinnamon and a pinch of sea salt, and mix until the nuts are thoroughly coated.
3. Transfer the nuts to the prepared baking tray and spread out in an even layer. Bake in the preheated oven for 7 minutes.
4. Remove from the oven and leave to cool completely on the tray. Break into 8 biscuit-sized clusters to serve.

These nut clusters will keep in an airtight container for 1–2 weeks.

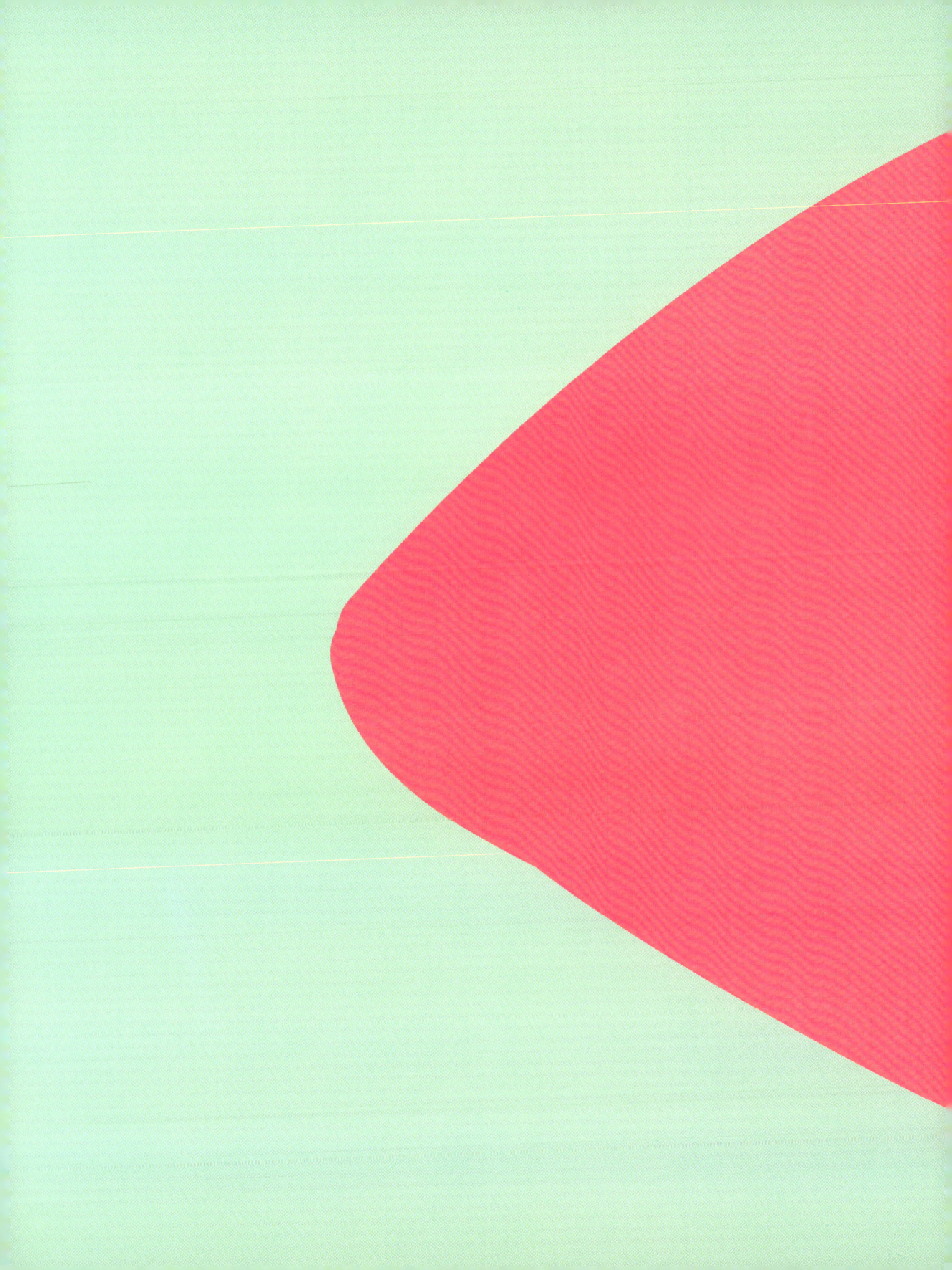

Dinner

Parmesan-crusted Fish Nuggets 120

Prawn Korma with Broccoli 122

Sneaky Spag Bol 125

Lamb and Harissa Burgers 126

Shepherd's Pie 129

Chicken with Bacon and Peas 130

Simple Chicken Stir Fry with Egg Noodles 132

Turkey and Quinoa Meatballs 135

Sausage Traybake 137

Pea and Pesto Courgetti Spaghetti 138

Dahl with Sweet Potato 141

Parmesan-crusted Fish Nuggets

This recipe is ideal for encouraging reluctant fish eaters! You can use cod or any firm white fish for this recipe. Frozen fillets work well, too. Just increase the cooking time by 2 minutes. Sautéed Smashed Peas (see page 146) would make a perfect companion to this delicious dish, as would the Air Fryer Sweet Potato Chips (see page 153).

Prep time 10 minutes | **Cook time** 8 minutes | **Serves** 2–4

Ingredients
4 tbsp polenta
40g Parmesan, finely grated
1 medium egg
1 tsp Dijon mustard
2 large skinless cod fillets, cut into cubes
Olive oil, for drizzling

Method
1. Line a baking tray with non-stick baking paper.
2. Mix the polenta in a bowl with the finely grated Parmesan and a pinch of salt. In another bowl, whisk the egg with the mustard.
3. Dip the fish pieces in the egg and mustard mixture, then into the polenta and Parmesan mixture, making sure the pieces are evenly coated. Transfer to the prepared baking tray. Scatter any leftover polenta and Parmesan mixture over the top.
4. Place the fish in an air fryer and drizzle with a little olive oil. Cook at 200°C for 8 minutes.

You could also cook these on the lined baking tray in an oven preheated to 220°C/ Fan 200°C/Gas 7 for 8–10 minutes.

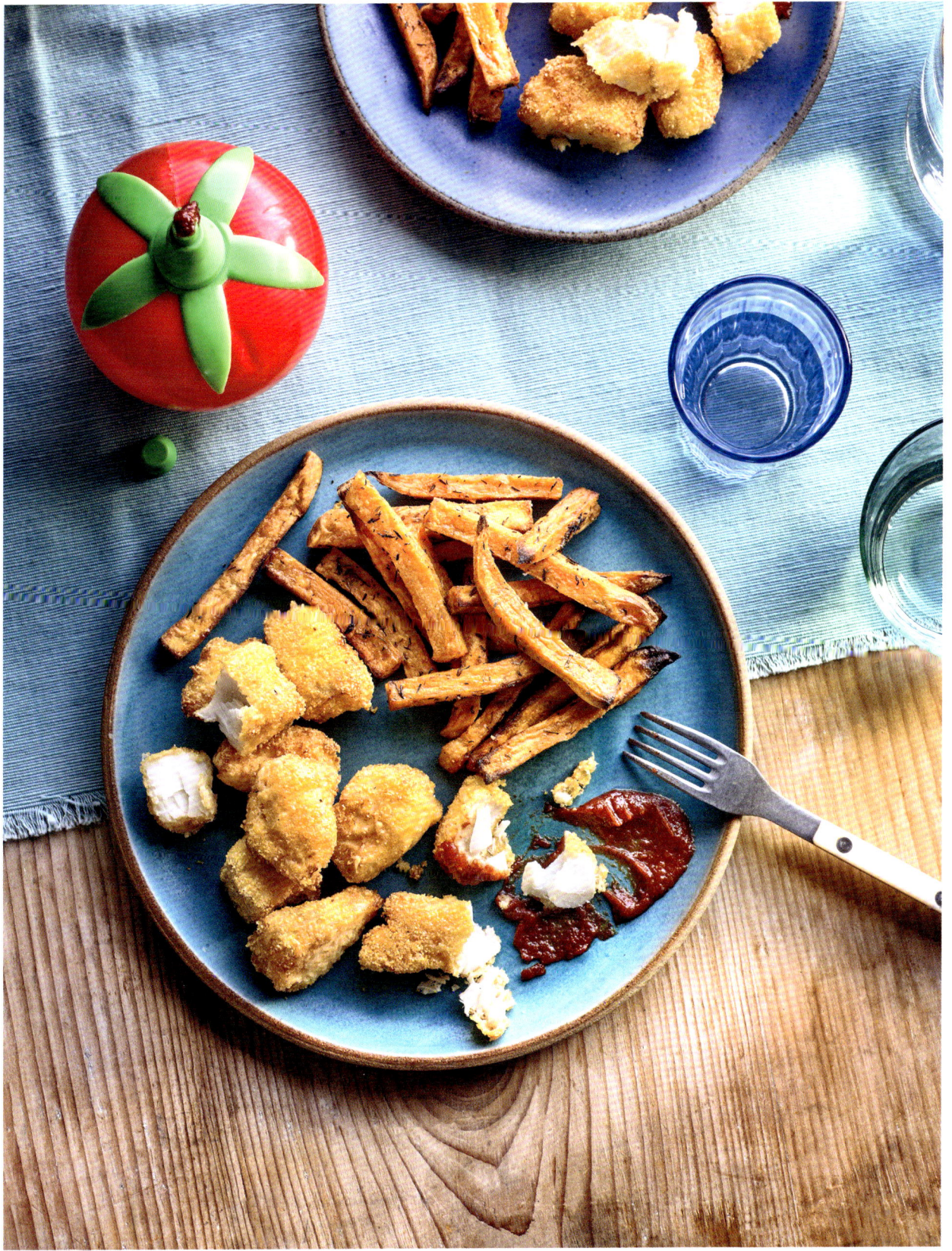

Prawn Korma with Broccoli

This mild curry is a great way to introduce children's palates to aromatic spices. Many of the ingredients can be found in the store cupboard or freezer. Use any veg you like and see the tip below on how to swap chicken for prawns. You might like to make your own curry powder by combining: 1 teaspoon ground cumin, 1 teaspoon ground coriander, ½ teaspoon ground turmeric and 1½ teaspoons garam masala.

Prep time 10 minutes | **Cook time** 15 minutes | **Serves** 4

Ingredients
2 tsp olive or coconut oil
1 small onion, finely chopped
1 garlic clove, finely chopped
1 tbsp curry powder
2 tbsp ground almonds
1 tbsp tomato purée
1 × 400g tin coconut milk
½ small head of broccoli, cut into small florets (about 160g)
450g frozen raw king prawns
4 tbsp full-fat Greek or natural yoghurt

Method
1. Heat the oil in a large non-stick frying pan over a medium heat. Add the onion and sauté for 3–4 minutes, stirring occasionally, until softened. Add the garlic and cook for 1 minute.
2. Stir in the curry powder, ground almonds and tomato purée, and cook for 1 minute. Add the coconut milk and broccoli, and bring to a simmer. Leave to bubble gently for 3–4 minutes.
3. Add the frozen prawns and bring back to a simmer. Cook for 2–3 minutes, until the prawns are pink and cooked through, and the broccoli is tender.
4. Remove from the heat, stir in the yoghurt and season with salt and freshly ground black pepper.
5. Serve with rice or Gluten-free Buckwheat Wraps (see page 101).

To replace the prawns with chicken, cut 3–4 chicken breasts into 2.5cm cubes and add them to the curry at the same time as the coconut milk. Simmer for 4 minutes, then add the broccoli and cook for a further 4 minutes.

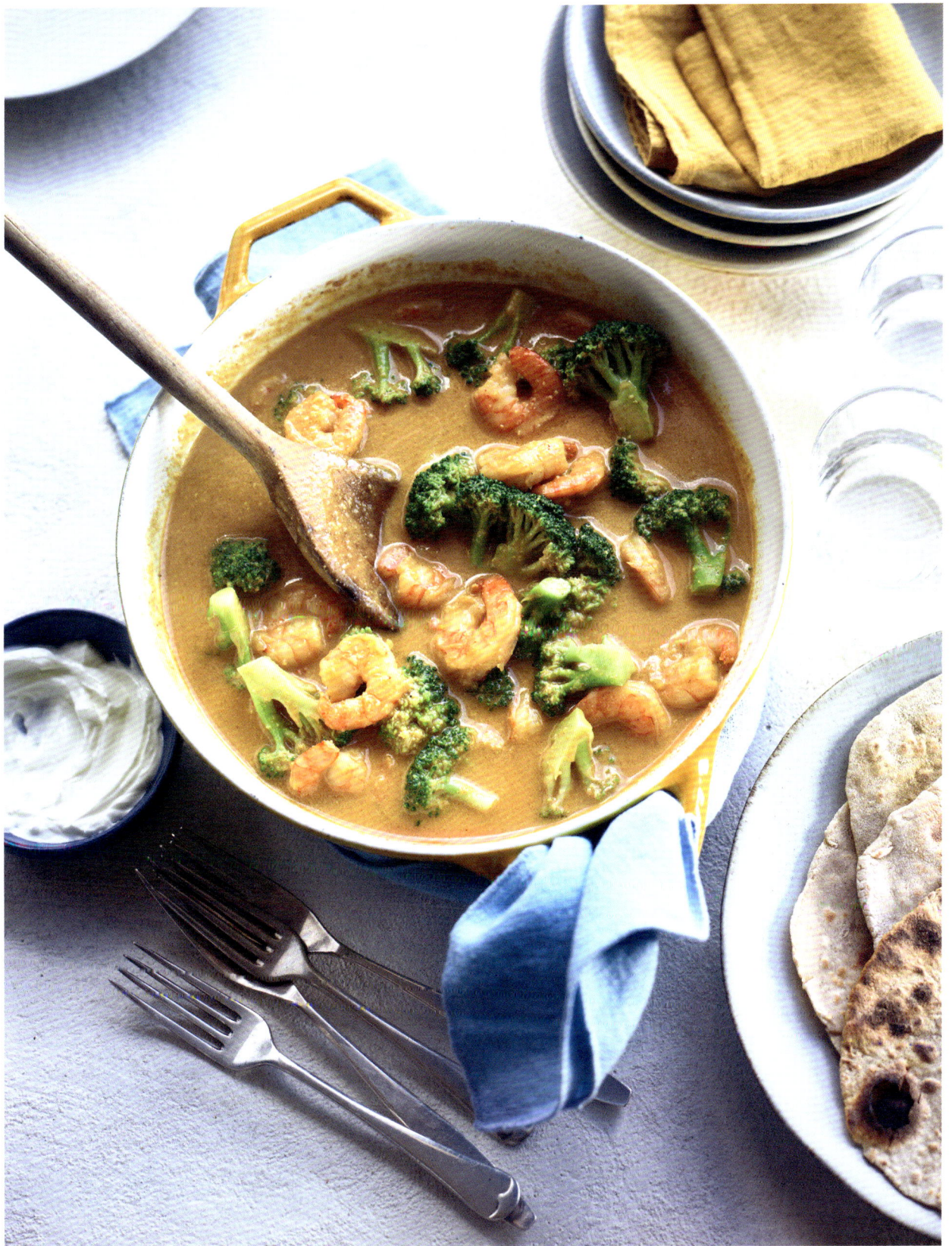

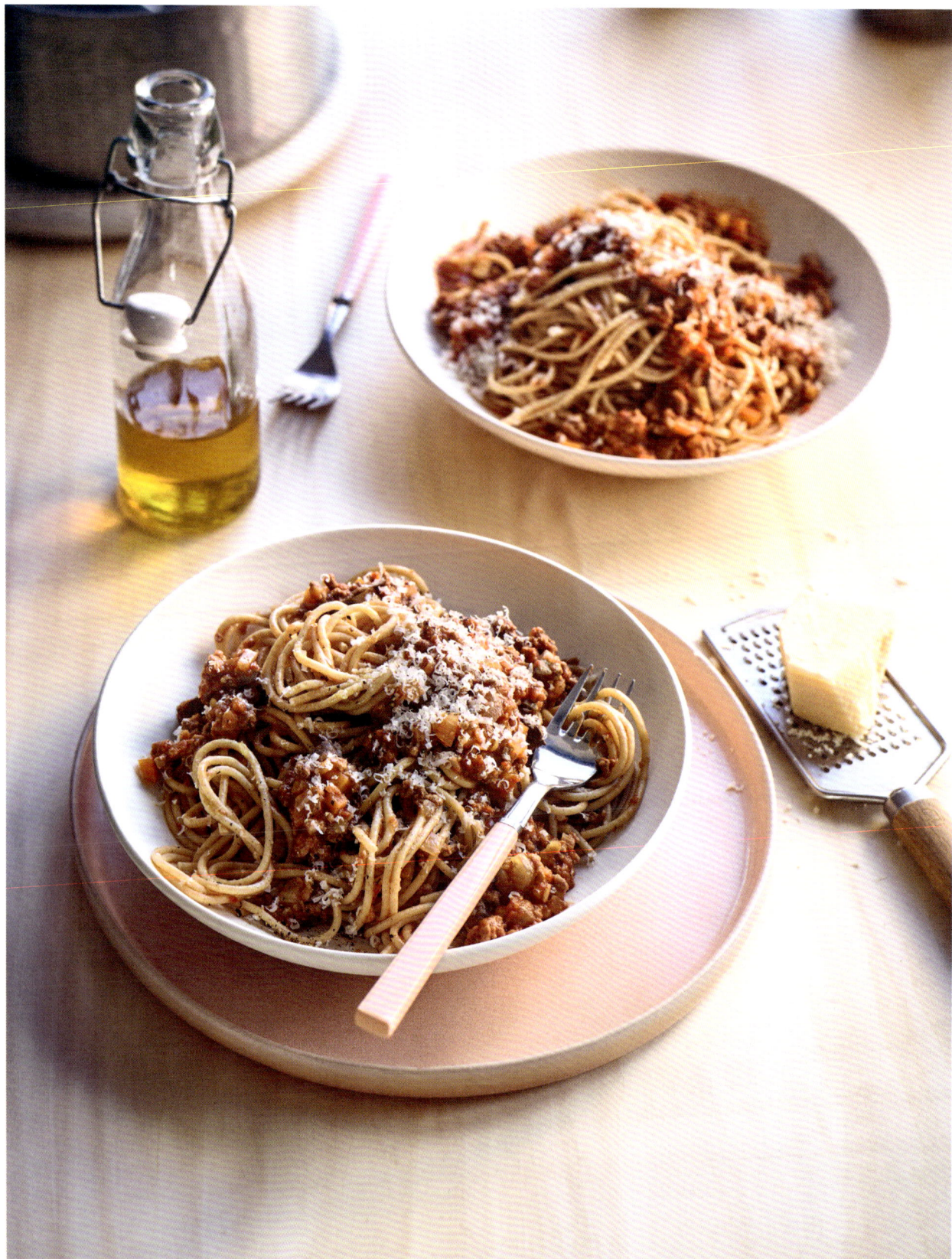

Sneaky Spag Bol

Here we sneak in some lentils and liver – both highly nutritious. Liver may seem like a strange addition but adds extra protein and nutrients, and gives a wonderful depth of flavour. Add spiralised courgette (zucchini) for even more vitamins, if you like.

Prep time 20 minutes | **Cook time** 50 minutes | Serves 4

Ingredients
3 tbsp olive oil
1 medium onion, finely chopped
1 carrot, finely chopped
2 celery sticks, trimmed and finely chopped
2 garlic cloves, finely chopped
2 tsp dried oregano
170g chicken livers, finely chopped
2 tbsp tomato purée
500g beef mince
5 tbsp red split lentils
2 × 400g tins chopped tomatoes
1 chicken or beef stock cube
450g wholegrain spaghetti
Parmesan or Cheddar, finely grated, to serve

Method
1. Heat 2 tablespoons of the olive oil in a large saucepan over a medium heat. Add the chopped vegetables and sauté with the garlic and thyme for 5–6 minutes, stirring occasionally, until softened. Transfer to a bowl.
2. Add the remaining olive oil to the pan, along with the chicken livers. Cook for 4–5 minutes, until very dark brown. Add the beef mince and break up with a wooden spoon. Cook for about 5 minutes, until browned all over.
3. Return the vegetables to the pan, along with the purée, lentils and chopped tomatoes. Half fill one empty tin with water and add to the pan. Crumble in the stock cube and stir. Cover, reduce the heat and simmer for 35 minutes. Season to taste with salt and black pepper.
4. Meanwhile, cook the pasta in a large pan of boiling salted water according to the packet instructions. Drain well.
5. Toss all the pasta with half of the sauce and serve topped with the grated cheese. Freeze the remaining sauce to use another day.

When bought in supermarkets, chicken livers can come in larger quantities than you need here. They freeze very well, though. As people get used to the flavour of liver, you can gradually increase the amount used in this Bolognese.

Lamb and Harissa Burgers

This is a burger with a mildly exotic flavour. The quantity of harissa used here is small, so the overall result is not at all spicy. The gherkins in the burgers provide health benefits as a fermented food – pickles are great for the gut and microbiome, and deliver a lovely, sweet and tangy flavour.

Prep time 20 minutes | **Cook time** 5 minutes | **Makes** 4

Ingredients
250g lamb mince
½ tsp ground cumin
1 tsp harissa
1 tbsp olive oil
1 large tomato, sliced
Baby gem lettuce
1 large gherkin, sliced (optional)
4 wholemeal baps or ciabatta buns

Method
1. In a bowl, mix the lamb mince, ground cumin, harissa and a pinch of salt and freshly ground black pepper. Divide into four and shape into burgers about 1cm thick.
2. Heat the oil in a large frying pan over a medium heat. When hot, add the lamb burgers and fry for 2½ minutes on each side. Remove from the pan and set aside to rest for 3 minutes.
3. Assemble the burgers by placing slices of tomato, some lettuce and gherkin in each bun. Serve with Cucumber in Yoghurt (see page 168).

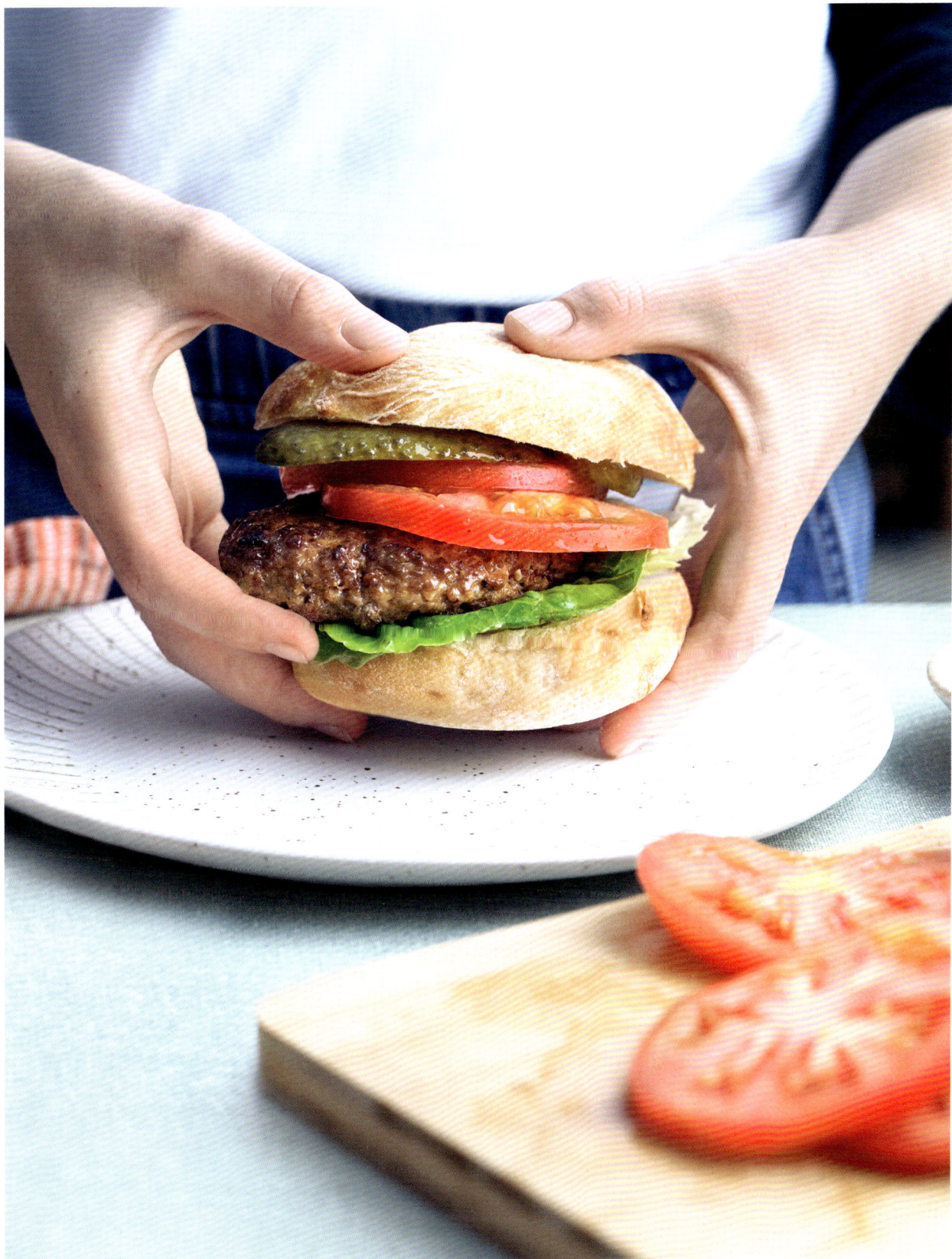

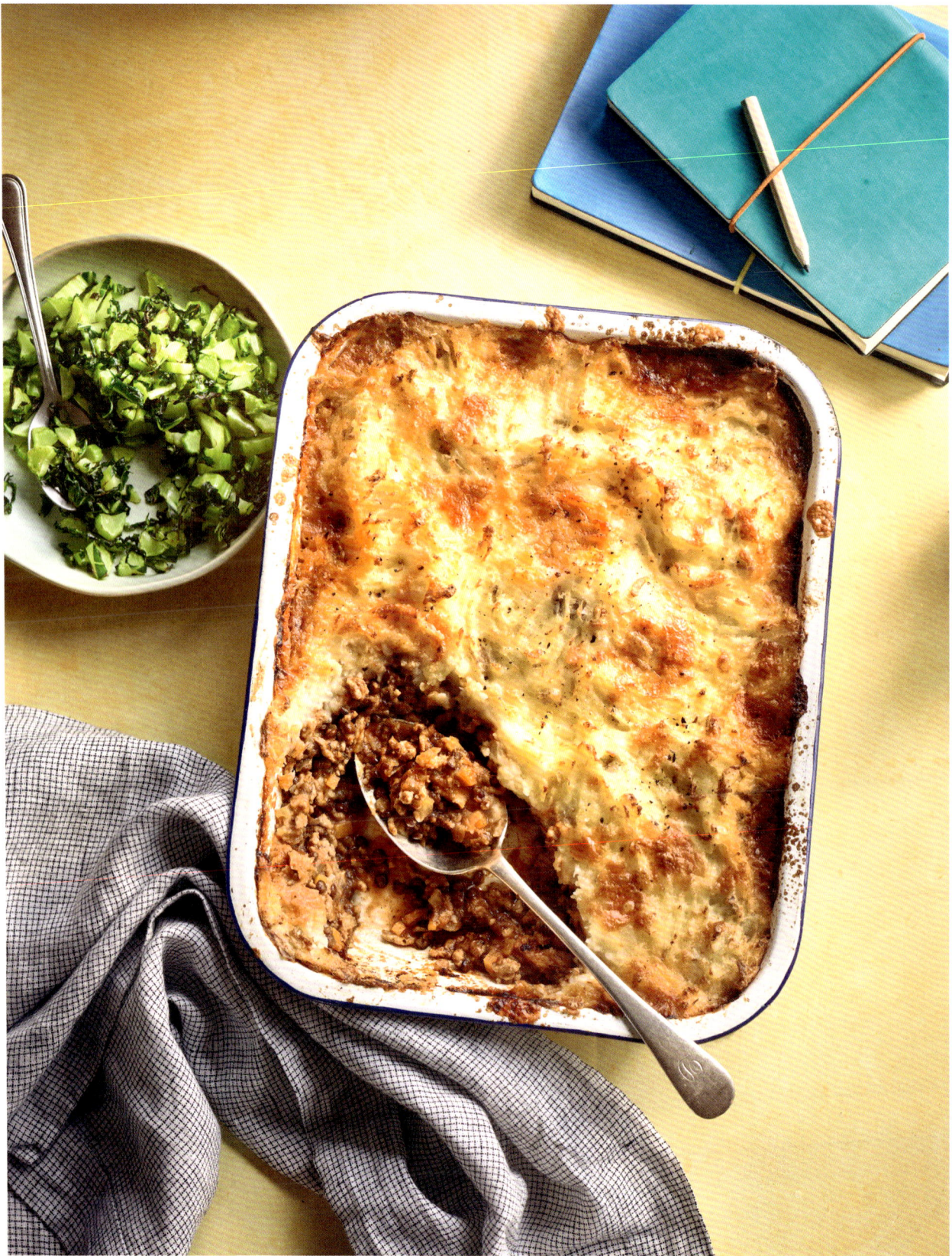

Shepherd's Pie

The potato skins provide extra fibre and nutrients here, while sneaking the lentils into the mince increases the amount of fibre and protein in this dish.

Prep time 35 minutes | **Cook time** 75 minutes | **Serves** 6 8

Ingredients
2 tbsp olive oil
1 large onion, finely diced
1 medium carrot, finely diced or grated
1 celery stick, trimmed and finely diced
1 tsp ground cinnamon
500g lamb mince
1 stock cube
500ml passata
1 tbsp mixed herbs
1 tbsp Worcestershire sauce (optional)
1 × 300g pouch ready-cooked lentils

Topping
650g potatoes, cut into 2cm dice (no need to peel)
325g cauliflower, cut into 2cm dice
60g butter or 3 tbsp olive oil
5–6 tbsp milk of choice
40g Cheddar, grated

Method
1. Heat the olive oil in a saucepan over a medium heat. Add the onion, carrot and celery and sweat for 4–5 minutes, stirring occasionally, until softened.
2. Increase the heat, add the cinnamon and lamb mince and cook, stirring frequently, until the meat is browned.
3. Crumble in the stock cube and add the passata, mixed herbs and Worcestershire sauce, if using. Add a splash of water, if needed, to cover the lamb with liquid. Cover with a lid and cook gently for 30 minutes.
4. Preheat the oven to 200°C/Fan 180°C/Gas 6.
5. Add the lentils to the saucepan and cook for another 10 minutes.
6. Meanwhile, in another medium pan, cook the potatoes and cauliflower in boiling salted water for about 15 minutes, until soft. Drain and stir in the butter or olive oil and the milk then mash vigorously, or give it a quick blitz with a stick blender. Season with salt and freshly ground black pepper.
7. Transfer the mince to an ovenproof dish, about 22 × 30cm, then top with the mash. Scatter with the grated cheese and bake in the preheated oven for 20–25 minutes, until golden brown.

Reserve the outer leaves of the cauliflower and finely chop them, then stir fry in some oil to serve as a vegetable side.

Chicken with Bacon and Peas

Warming, comforting, budget-friendly and full of flavour – this is perfect comfort food. It's also high in protein. If you prefer, you could use 100g diced chorizo instead of the bacon lardons.

Prep time 10 minutes | **Cook time** 50 minutes | **Serves** 4

Ingredients
1 tbsp olive oil
4 chicken legs (about 1kg)
200g bacon lardons or strips
1 small onion, finely chopped
2 garlic cloves, finely chopped
4 sprigs of thyme, leaves picked, or 2 tsp dried thyme
1 tbsp plain flour
500ml chicken stock
200g frozen peas
60g crème fraîche

Method
1. Preheat the oven to 170°C/Fan 150°C/Gas 3½.
2. Heat the olive oil in a large casserole over a medium heat. Add the chicken and brown, skin side down, for 5 minutes. Remove from the pan and set aside.
3. Add the bacon to the pan and fry for 2–3 minutes, until browned and crispy. Remove from the pan and set aside with the chicken.
4. Add the onion to the pan and sauté for 2–3 minutes, until softened, then stir in the garlic and thyme. Cook for 1 minute more.
5. Stir in the flour, then return the bacon to the pan and pour in the stock. Stir over the heat until thickened. Return the chicken to the pan, pushing it down a little so it is covered by the stock. Bring to the boil, then cover with a lid and transfer to the preheated oven for 40 minutes. Add the peas for the last 5 minutes of the cooking time.
6. Remove the casserole from the oven and stir in the crème fraîche. Serve with tenderstem broccoli (broccolini) on the side.

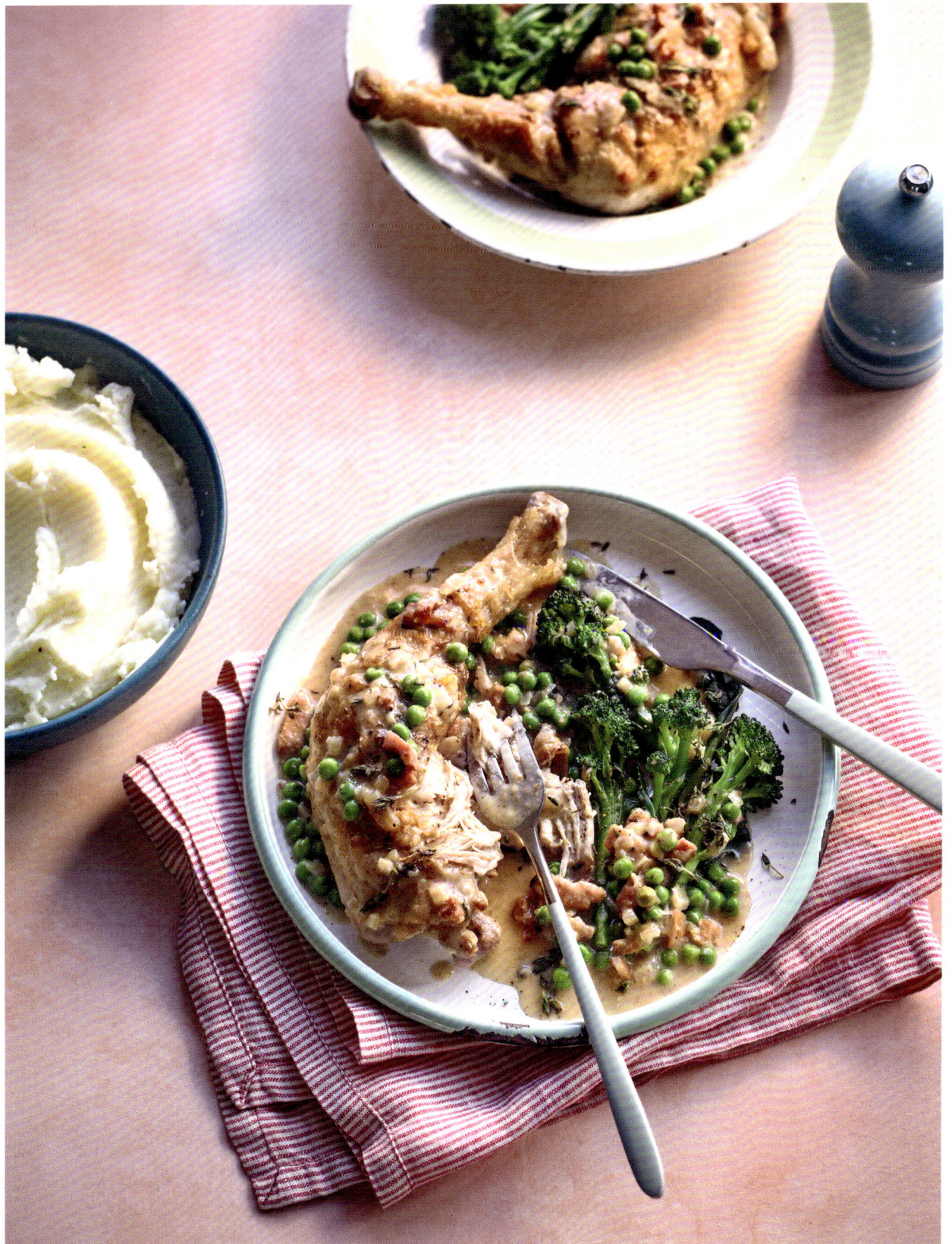

Simple Chicken Stir Fry with Egg Noodles

Pak choi is high in nutrients and an excellent source of gut-friendly soluble fibre. Some supermarkets sell ready-cooked egg noodles, which are more convenient than dried. To make this recipe vegetarian, replace the chicken with tofu or tempeh.

Prep time 15 minutes, plus marinating time | **Cook time** 20 minutes | **Serves** 4

Ingredients
500g skinless, boneless chicken thighs, sliced into thin strips
4 tbsp soy sauce or tamari
3 tbsp olive or coconut oil
1 medium onion, finely diced
2 red peppers (capsicums), deseeded and cut into 2cm dice
2 heads of pak choi, finely shredded
250g dried egg noodles
½ tbsp sesame oil (optional)
½ tsp chilli flakes (optional)

Method
1. Place the chicken in a large shallow dish and pour in the soy sauce. Season with ground black pepper and leave to marinate for 15 minutes.
2. Heat 1 tablespoon of the oil in a wok or large non-stick frying pan over a high heat. When it is very hot and the oil begins to smoke, add half the chicken and stir fry for 5–6 minutes, until golden and cooked through. Remove from the pan and repeat with another tablespoon of oil and the remaining chicken. Remove the chicken from the pan and keep warm.
3. Add the remaining oil to the pan and, when hot, add the onion and peppers (capsicums) and stir fry for about 3 minutes, until soft but still retaining some bite. Reduce the heat and add the pak choi and any remaining marinade from the chicken. Cook for 2 minutes, until wilted. Return the chicken to the pan and toss to combine. Remove from the heat, cover and keep warm.
4. Meanwhile, cook the noodles according to packet instructions. Drain, reserving 2 tablespoons of the cooking water.
5. Add the noodles and reserved water to the pan with the chicken and vegetables. Dress with the sesame oil and chilli flakes, if using, and toss well to combine. Serve immediately.

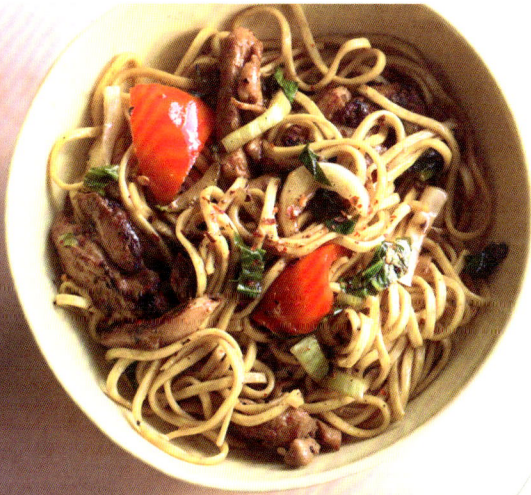

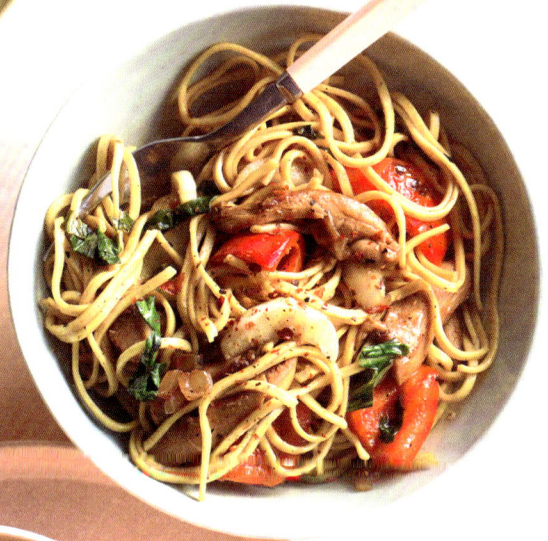

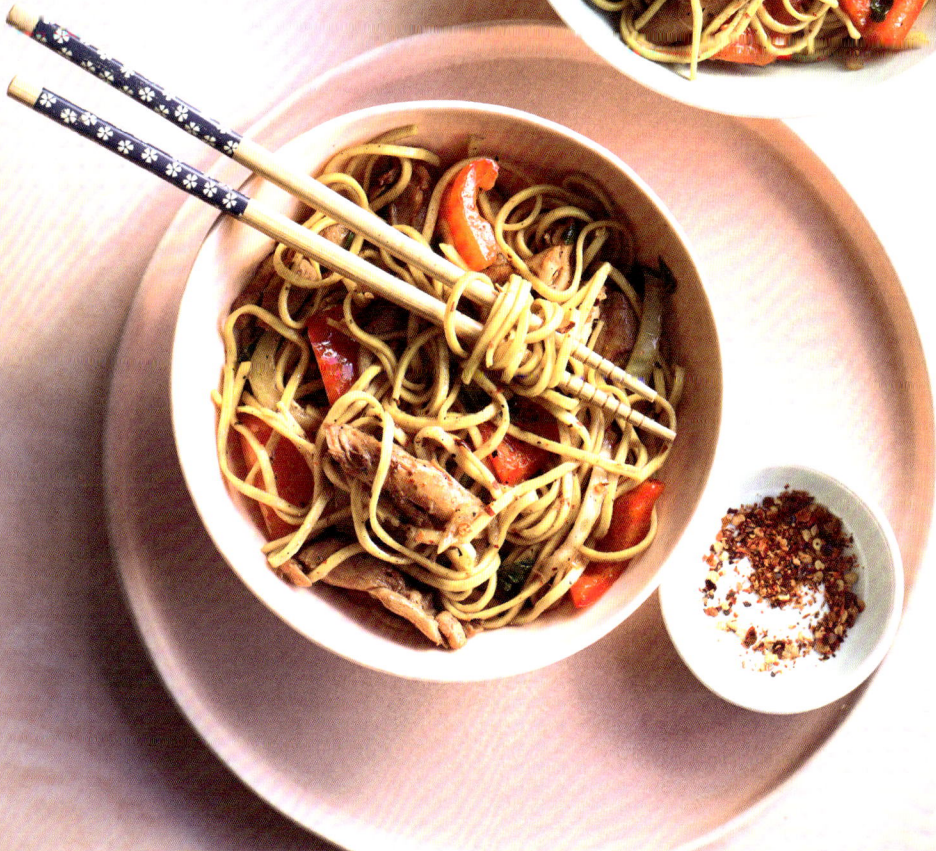

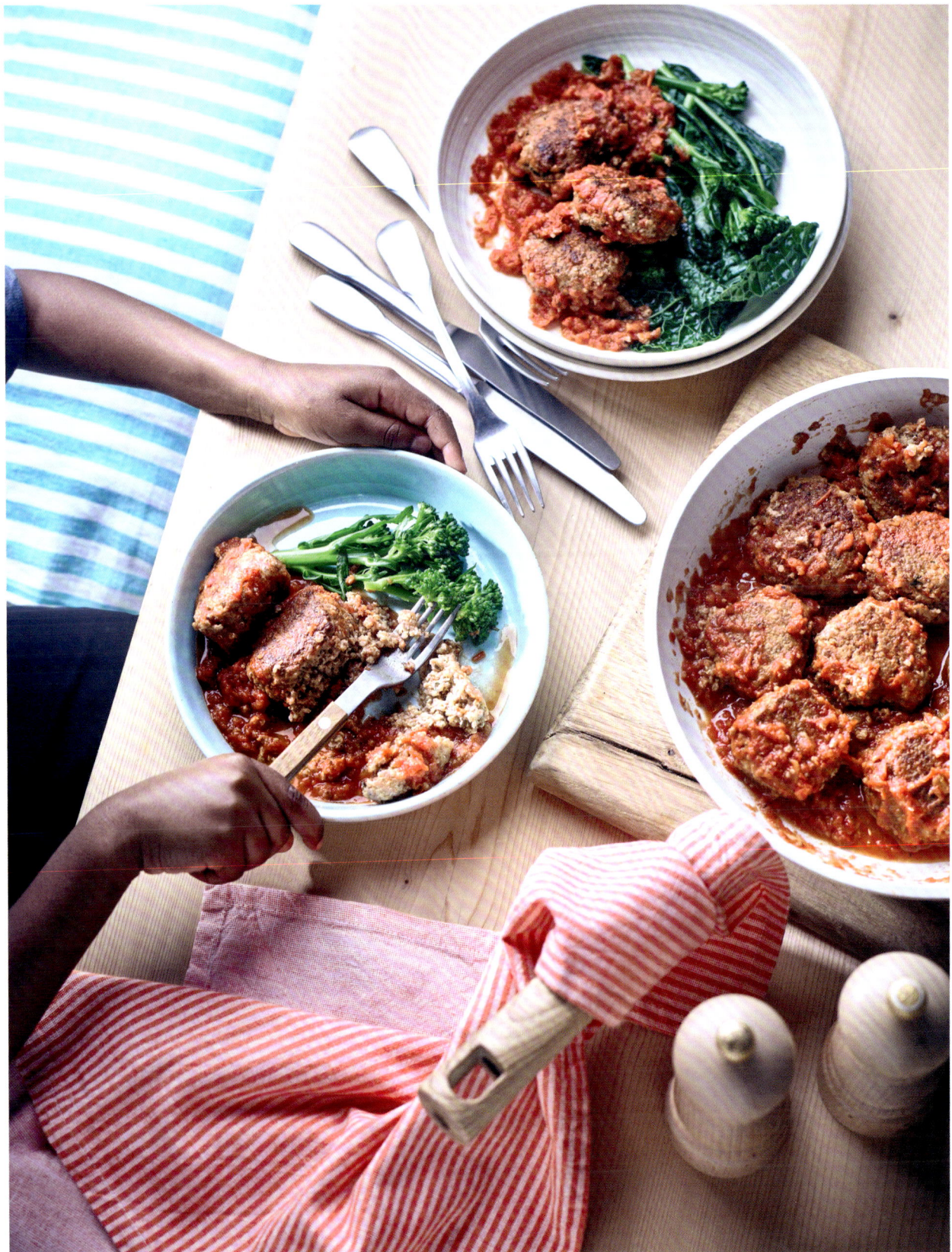

Turkey and Quinoa Meatballs

The portions here are generous. If you feel there are too many meatballs for the size of your family, simply freeze what you don't need and use them another time. If any of your children are averse to chunky sauces, blitz the sauce before adding the meatballs back in – just be careful as the sauce will be hot. The Six Veg Tomato Sauce (see page 164) would also work perfectly here if you have some.

Prep time 15 minutes | **Cook time** 25 minutes | **Serves** 4–6

Ingredients
500g turkey thigh mince
100g cooked quinoa
1 tbsp wholemeal or spelt flour
1 medium egg
3 tbsp sun-dried tomato pesto
3 sprigs of basil, leaves picked and finely chopped (optional)
2 tbsp olive oil, plus extra for drizzling
1 × 400g tin chopped tomatoes
25g Parmesan, finely grated, to garnish (optional)

Method
1. Place the turkey thigh mince, quinoa, flour, egg, 2 tablespoons of the pesto and the basil, if using, in a large bowl. Season with salt and freshly ground black pepper and use a wooden spoon to mix everything together. Use damp hands to create 16 golf-ball-sized meatballs.
2. Heat the oil in a large non-stick frying pan with a lid over a medium heat. Add the meatballs and fry for 3 minutes on each side, until golden brown. You may need to do this in batches. Remove them from the pan and set aside.
3. Pour the tinned tomatoes into the unwashed pan and half fill the empty tin with water. Add this to the pan along with the remaining pesto and a drizzle of olive oil. Increase the heat and simmer vigorously for 2–3 minutes, until thickened. Season to taste.
4. Return the meatballs to the pan and cover with the lid. Reduce the heat and simmer for 15 minutes.
5. Serve the meatballs with broccoli or steamed greens and garnish with Parmesan, if using.

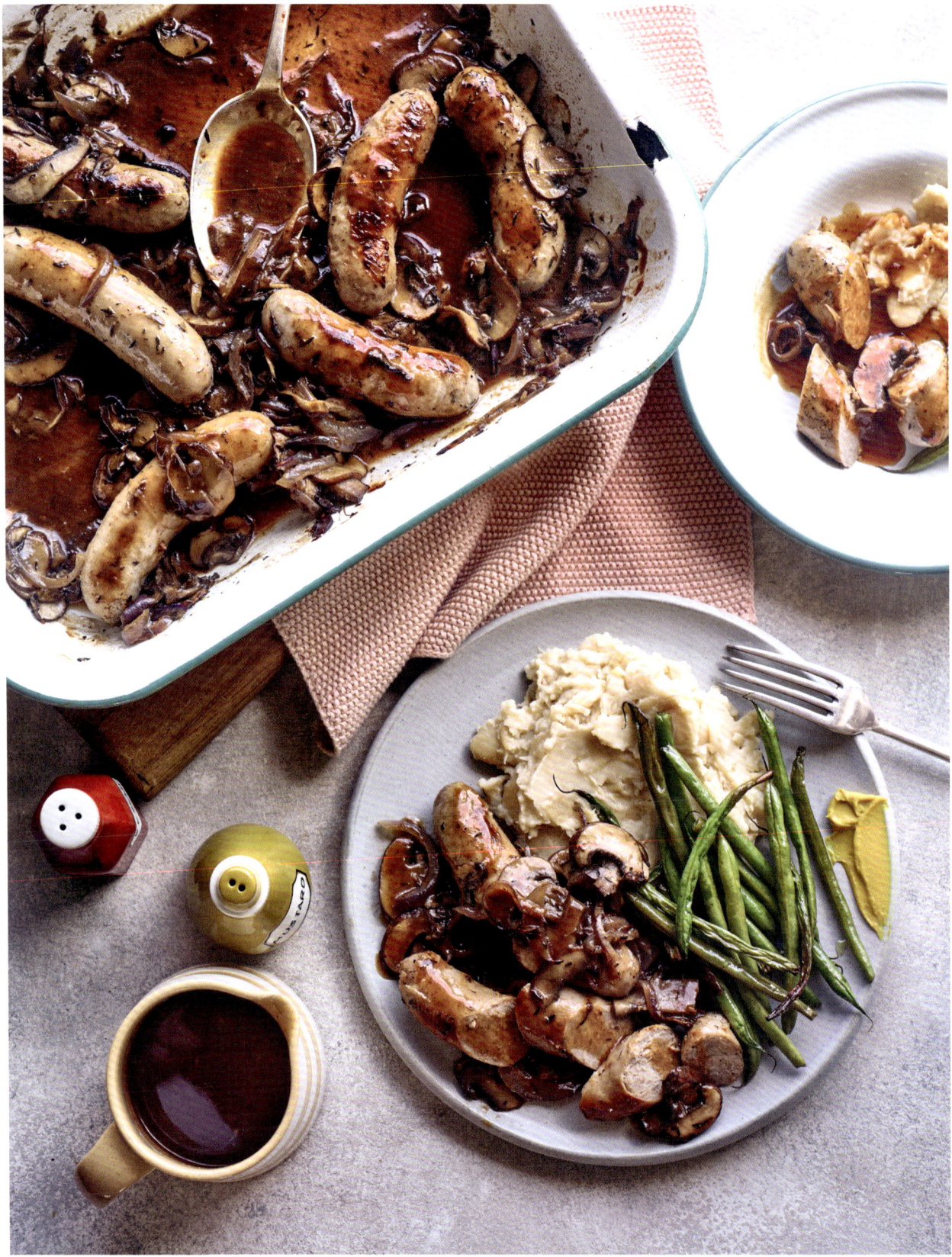

Sausage Traybake

This is a quick and easy sausage supper with a lovely gravy.

Prep time 10 minutes | **Cook time** 35 minutes | **Serves** 4

Ingredients
1 red onion, sliced
250g chestnut or Swiss Brown mushrooms, finely sliced
1 tsp dried thyme
1½ tbsp olive oil
8 sausages (about 500g)
300ml chicken stock
2 tbsp brown sauce or 1 tbsp Worcestershire sauce
1 tsp cornflour

Method
1. Preheat the oven to 190°C/Fan 170°C/Gas 5.
2. Arrange the onion and mushrooms in the base of a medium roasting tin (roughly 23 × 33cm). Scatter over the thyme and drizzle with the olive oil. Place the sausages on top, then pour 100ml of the stock into the tin. Roast in the preheated oven for 30 minutes, turning the sausages halfway through.
3. Take the tin out of the oven and remove the sausages. Set them aside and keep warm. Pour the remaining stock into the tin and add the brown sauce or Worcestershire sauce. Stir well.
4. In a small bowl, mix the cornflour with 1 tablespoon water until smooth, then stir this into the gravy. Return the tin to the oven for 5 minutes, or until the gravy has thickened. Season to taste.
5. Serve the sausages topped with the gravy and some Garlicky Green Beans (see page 157) and mashed butter beans on the side.

Pea and Pesto Courgetti Spaghetti

Recipe writer Kathryn has been making this pesto since her children were little and they turn away from shop-bought varieties having got used to the taste of something fresher. Think of this as more than a pasta sauce – it can be served with sliced vegetables as a snack or used in sandwiches and wraps. Adding spiralised courgettes (zucchini) to pasta is a fun way to introduce some extra veg. In the absence of a spiraliser, you could finely chop or grate the courgette (zucchini) instead.

Prep time 15 minutes | **Cook time** 8–10 minutes | **Serves** 2

Ingredients
80g wholegrain spaghetti
1 small courgette (zucchini), spiralised
100g feta, crumbled

For the pea and basil pesto
4 sprigs of basil, leaves picked
20g Parmesan, roughly chopped
20g cashew nuts or blanched almonds
70g frozen peas, defrosted
2 tbsp olive oil

Method
1. To make the pesto, place all the ingredients in a jug or deep bowl with 1 tablespoon of water and use a stick blender to blitz until smooth. Season to taste with salt and freshly ground black pepper.
2. Cook the spaghetti in a large pan of boiling salted water according to the packet instructions. Add the courgette (zucchini) for the last minute of cooking. Drain and reserve 2 tablespoons of the cooking water.
3. Toss the pasta with the pesto, adding some of the cooking water to loosen, if necessary.
4. Top with the feta and serve straight away.

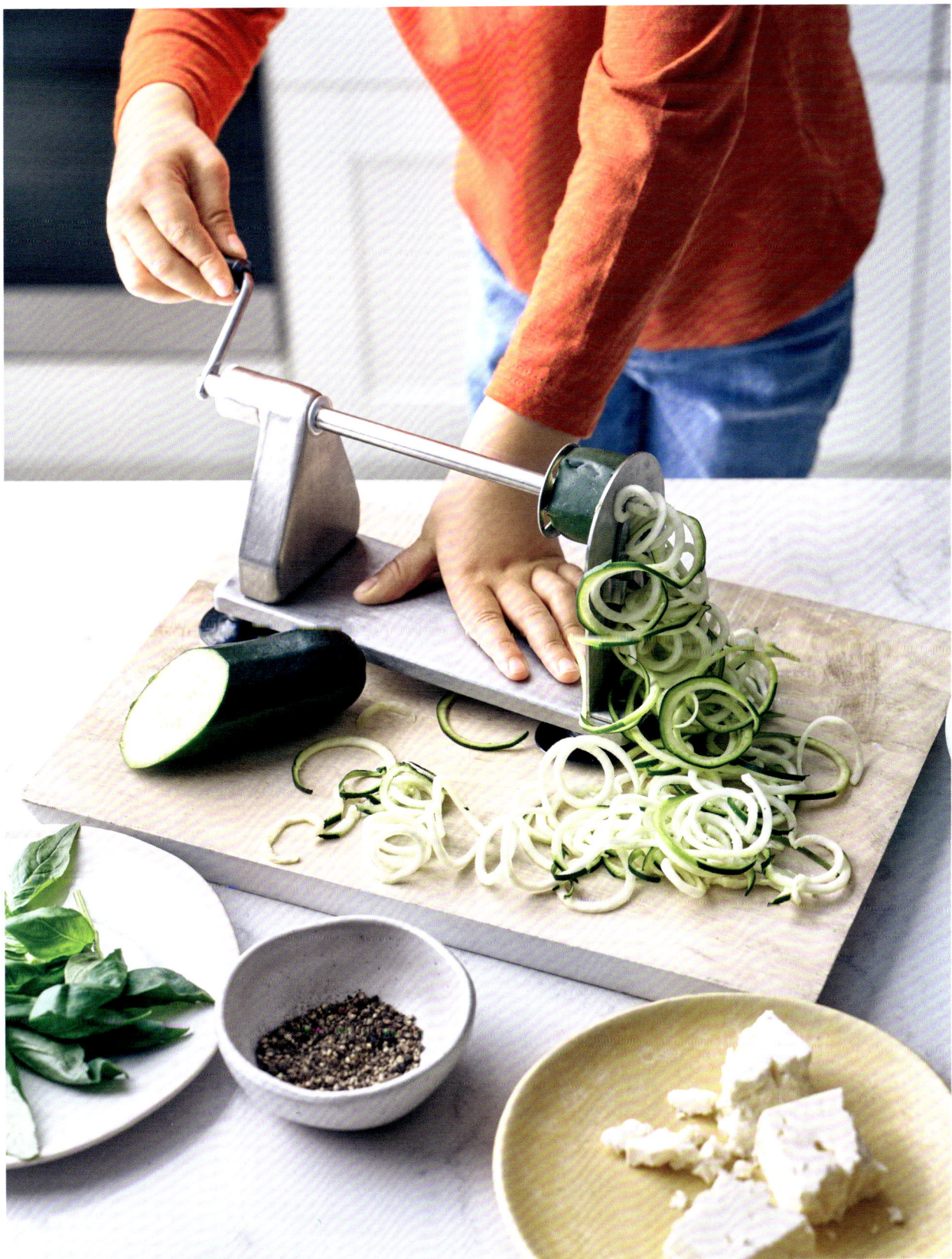

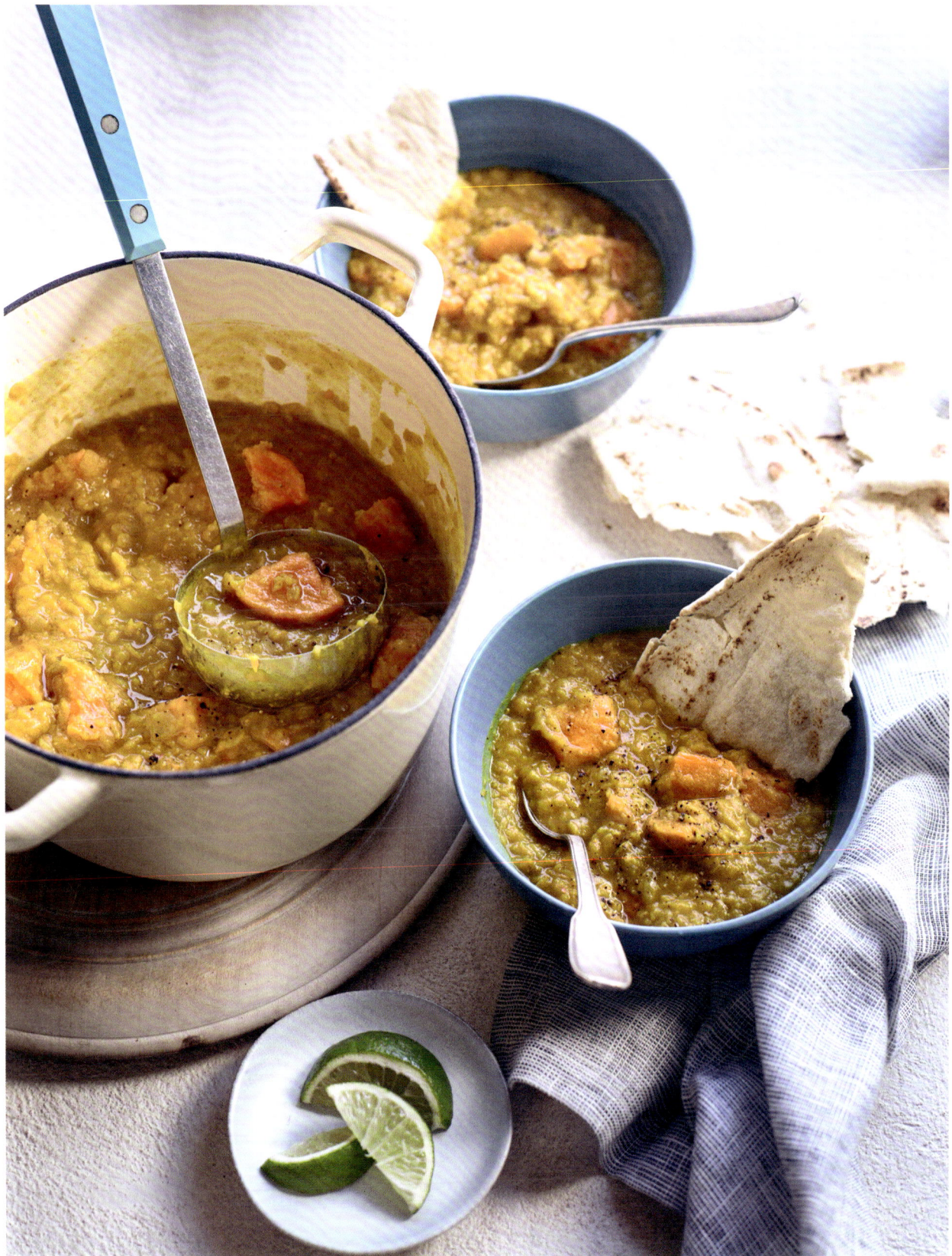

Dahl with Sweet Potato

Dhal is one of my favourite easy and versatile dishes. You can add extra flavours, more veg or protein, or turn it into a soup simply by loosening it with a little more water, which I often do. It also makes a fabulous and flavourful side dish. The microbes in your gut will think it's Christmas come early.

Prep time 10 minutes | **Cook time** 25 minutes | **Serves** 4

Ingredients
1 medium onion, finely chopped
3 tbsp olive oil
1 tsp mild curry powder
1 tsp ground turmeric
1 tsp finely chopped fresh ginger (or use ½ tsp ground ginger)
1 large sweet potato, peeled and cut into 2cm dice
200g red split lentils
1 vegetable stock cube
2 bay leaves (optional)
Juice of ½ lime

Method
1. In a medium saucepan or casserole with a lid, sauté the onion in the oil over a medium heat for 3–4 minutes, stirring occasionally.
2. Add the spices, ginger, sweet potato and red lentils, and pour in 500ml water. Crumble in the stock cube, add the bay leaves, if using, and mix well. Reduce the heat, cover and simmer for 20 minutes, stirring from time to time, until the sweet potato is tender and the lentils cooked through. Add a splash more water, if needed, as it thickens.
3. Remove from the heat, stir in the lime juice, and season with lots of freshly ground black pepper and a pinch of salt.
4. Serve on its own or with some paneer or feta crumbled on top.

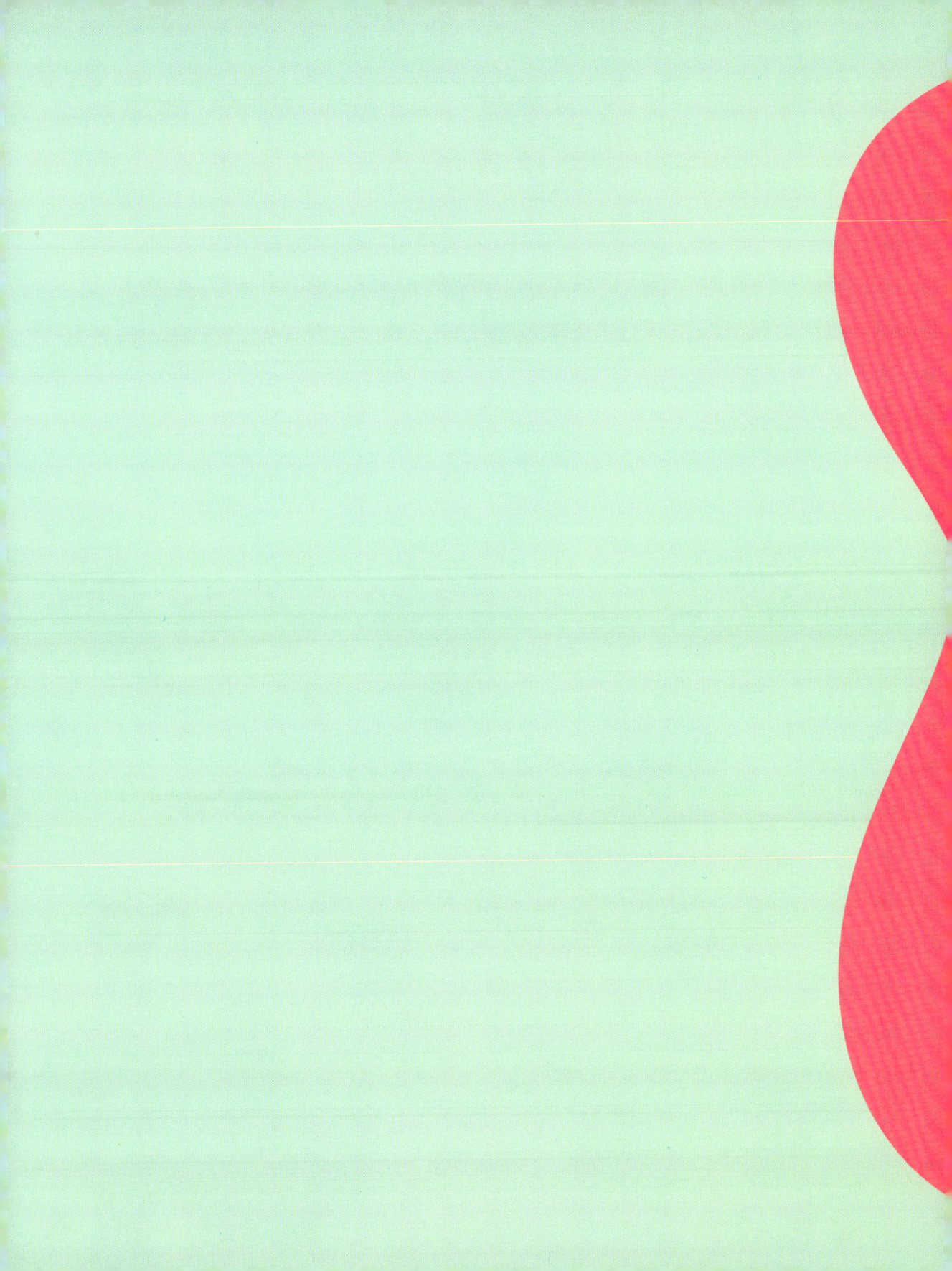

Veggie sides

Roasted Pesto and Parmesan Pumpkin

The Parmesan, with its umami flavour, creates a deliciously crispy crust on the roasted pumpkin, which should go down a treat with little ones. Mild curry powder would be a fantastic flavour addition here, if you want to try something different – add ½ teaspoon curry powder to the olive oil.

Prep time 5 minutes | **Cook time** 25 minutes | **Serves** 4

Ingredients
1½ tsp sun-dried tomato pesto
2 tbsp olive oil
350g frozen butternut pumpkin (squash)
40g Parmesan, finely grated

Method
1. Preheat the oven to 220°C/Fan 200°C/Gas 7 and line a large baking tray with non-stick baking paper.
2. In a large bowl, mix the pesto and olive oil with a pinch of salt, then add the pumpkin (squash) and toss to coat. Separate any pieces of frozen pumpkin (squash) that are stuck together.
3. Spread out in a single layer on the prepared baking tray and roast in the preheated oven for 20 minutes.
4. Carefully remove the tray from the oven, scatter the Parmesan all over, and a little black pepper then return it to the oven to roast for a further 5 minutes.
5. Leave to cool slightly before serving.

You can use fresh butternut pumpkin (squash) here – just peel the pumpkin and cut the flesh into 2cm cubes.

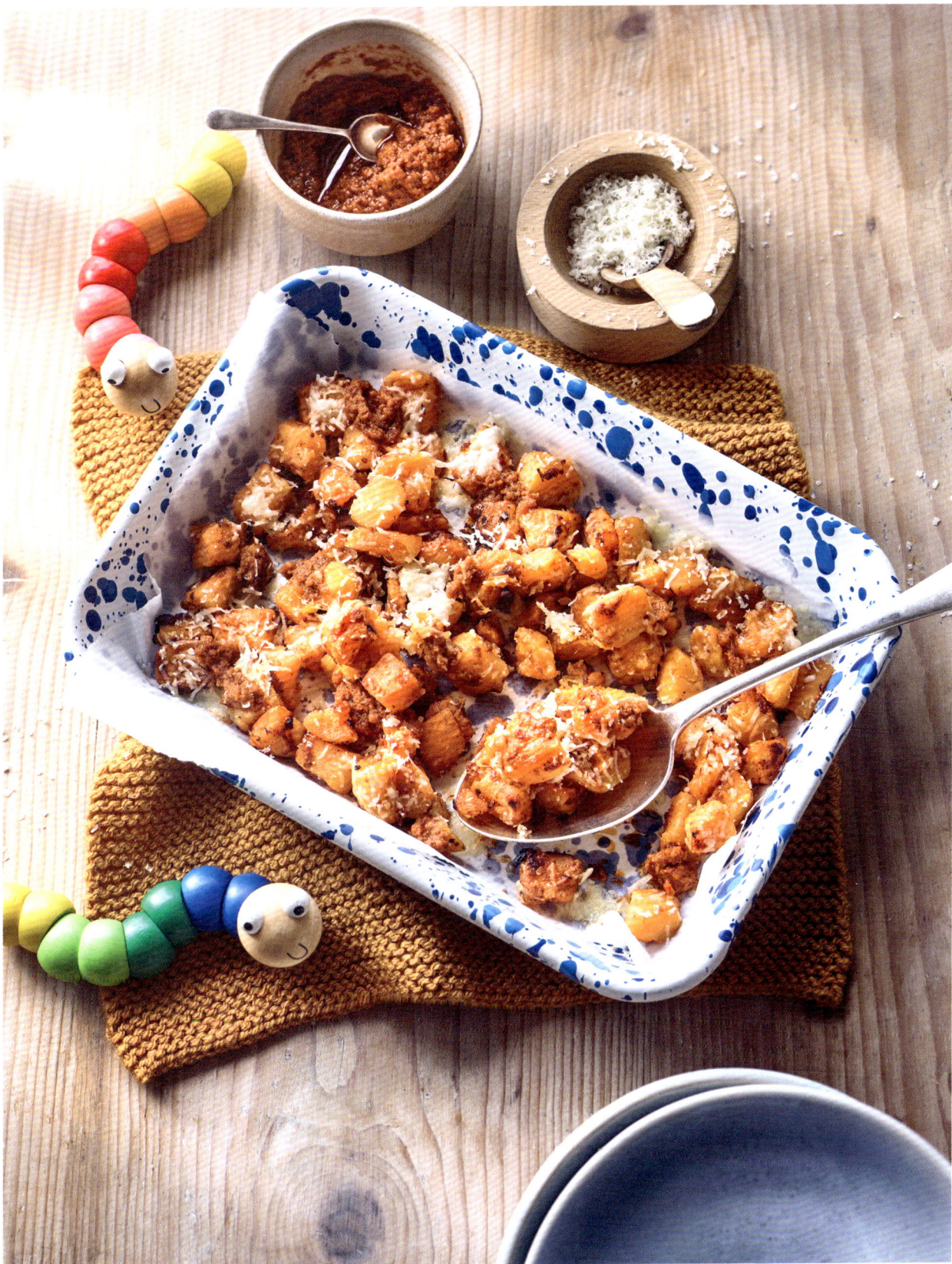

Sautéed Smashed Peas

Trying to keep peas on a fork, let alone on the plate, can be a challenge. By gently crushing them, they are easier to eat and seem tastier, too, especially with the sweet taste of the garlic. Some finely chopped mint would also make a lovely addition. You can make this ahead of time and just heat it up. This is still one of my favourite ways to enjoy peas.

Prep time 5 minutes | **Cook time** 7 minutes | **Serves** 4

Ingredients
200g frozen peas
Boiling water
1½ tbsp olive oil
½ small onion, finely chopped
1 small garlic clove, finely chopped (optional)

Method
1. Place the frozen peas in a bowl and cover with boiling water to defrost. Set aside.
2. Heat the oil in a frying pan over a medium heat. Add the onion and sauté for 3–4 minutes, until softened, stirring often to stop it from catching and burning. Add the garlic, if using, and cook for 1 minute more.
3. Remove the pan from the heat, drain the peas and add them to the pan. Return to the heat and sauté until the peas are hot.
4. Use a potato masher to smash the peas slightly, season with salt and freshly ground black pepper and serve.

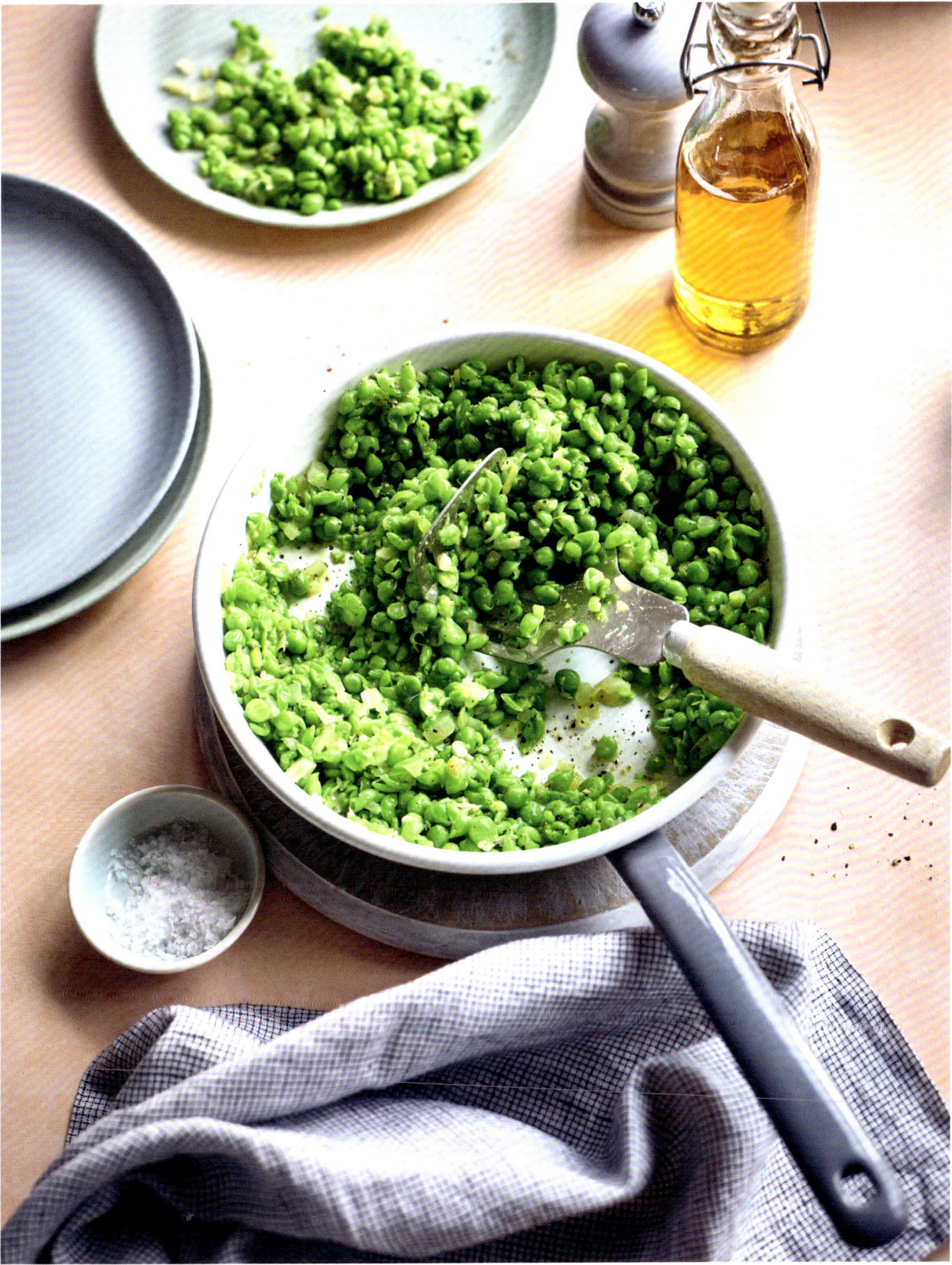

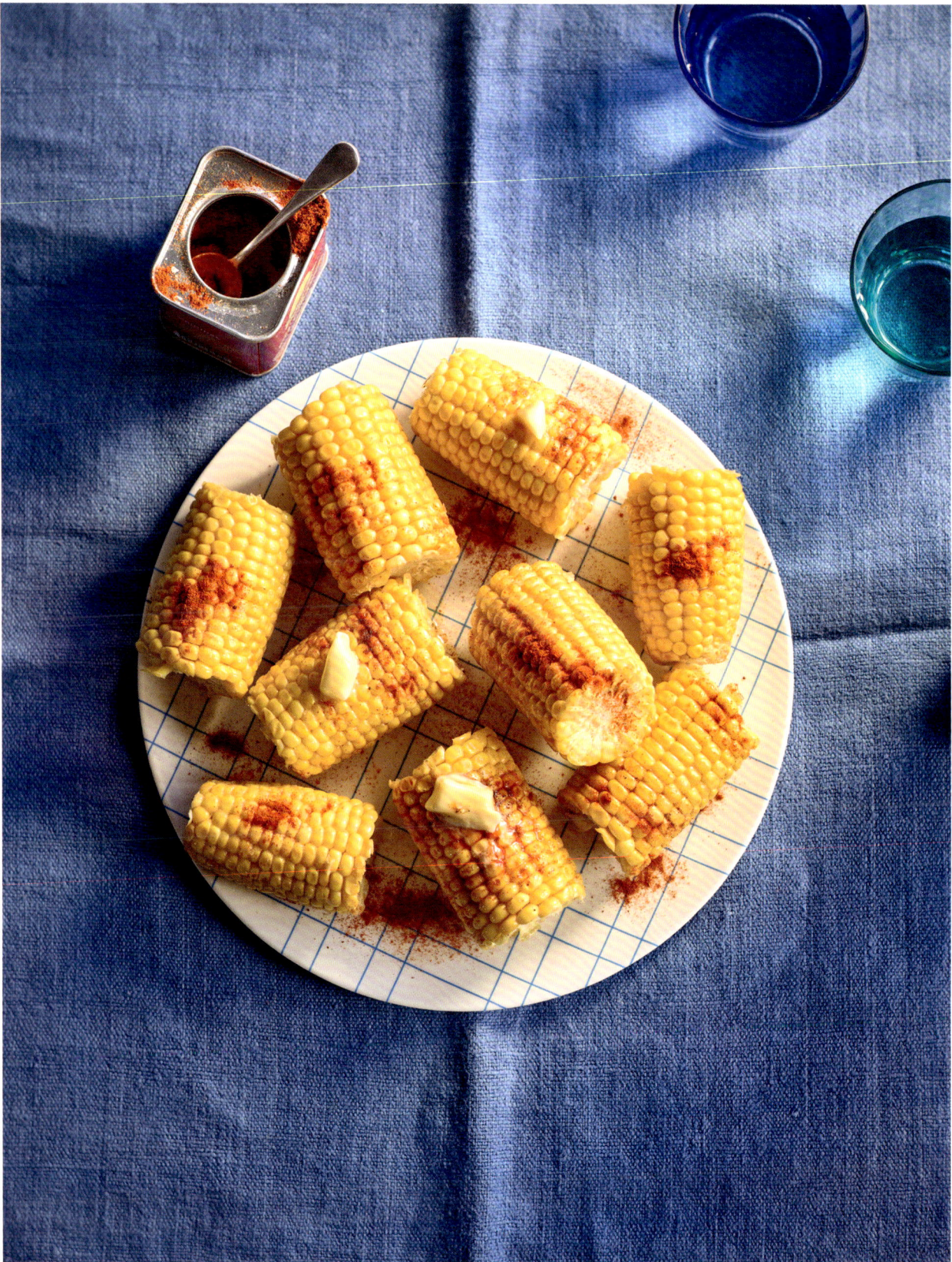

Sweetcorn with Butter and Paprika

These are great source of fibre. You can buy bags of frozen corn on the cob, which are a fantastic standby to have in your freezer.

Prep time 3 minutes | **Cook time** 8 minutes | **Serves** 4

Ingredients
4 small corn on the cob
Boiling water
1 tbsp butter or olive oil
Pinch of paprika

Method
1. Place the corn in a medium saucepan and cover with boiling water. Set the saucepan over a medium heat and simmer for 8 minutes. Drain and set aside to cool slightly.
2. Toss with the butter or olive oil, and season with a pinch of salt. Serve dusted with the paprika.

Baked Spinach with Parmesan

This dish combines the creaminess of spinach and cheese to make a tasty, umami-flavoured bake. You could add some crumbled feta and finely chopped roasted red peppers (capsicums), if you like, to make this dish more of a main event and even more delicious.

Prep time 15 minutes | **Cook time** 20 minutes | **Serves** 4

Ingredients
Butter or olive oil, for greasing
500g frozen spinach, defrosted
2 medium eggs
200g crème fraîche
50g Parmesan, finely grated
½ tsp ground nutmeg

Method
1. Preheat the oven to 200°C/Fan 180°C/Gas 6 and grease a 13 × 18cm roasting or enamel dish with a little butter or olive oil and set aside.
2. Squeeze as much water from the defrosted spinach as possible, then place in a bowl with the eggs, crème fraîche, Parmesan and nutmeg. Season with salt and a generous pinch of freshly ground black pepper and mix to combine. Make sure there are no clumps of spinach.
3. Transfer to the prepared dish and bake in the preheated oven for 20 minutes, or until just set.
4. Serve immediately, or leave to cool and refrigerate to enjoy later as a cold snack or light lunch.

You can also turn this into muffins. Spoon the mixture into silicone muffin cases and bake as above, reducing the cooking time to 10–15 minutes.

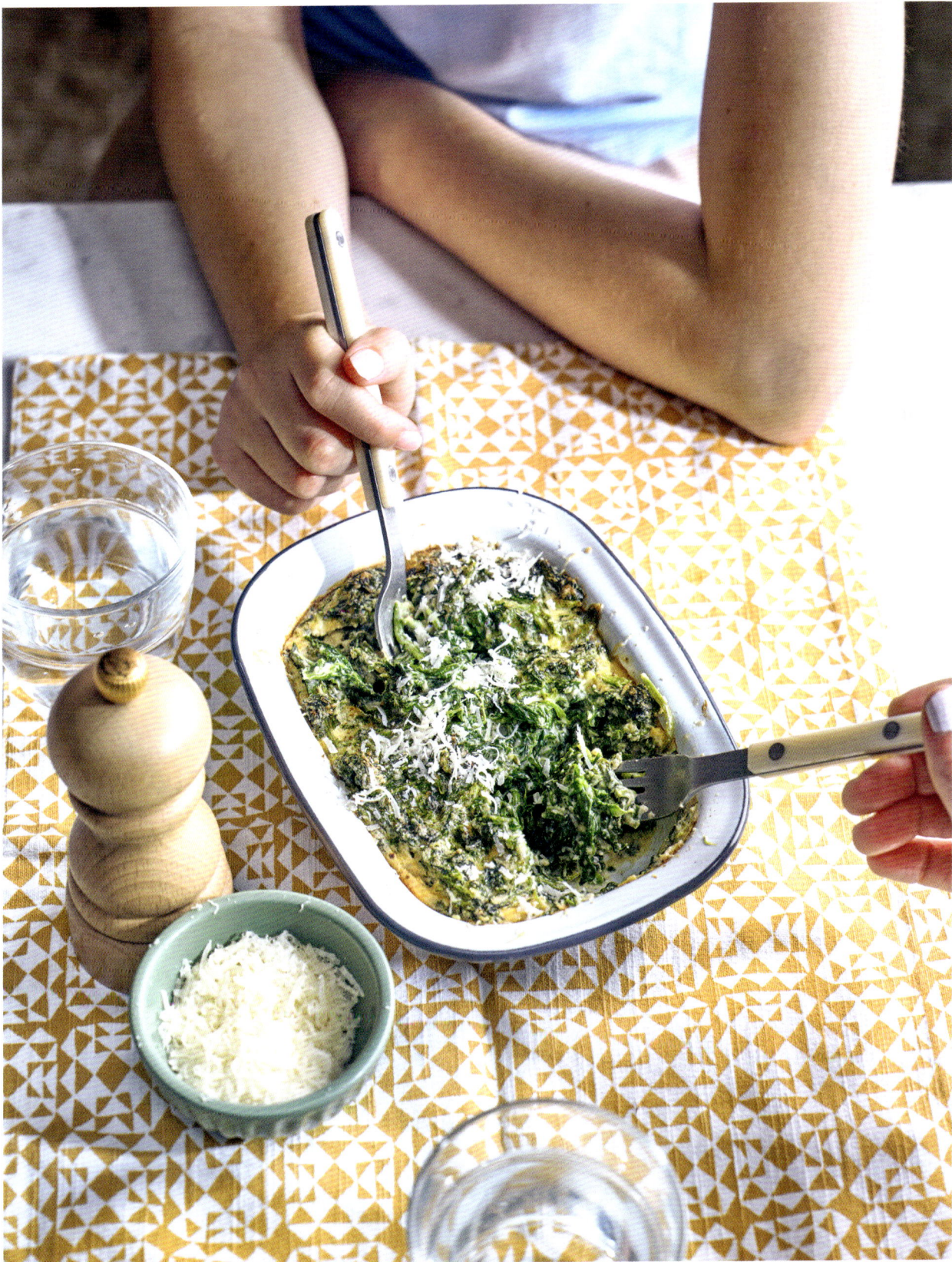

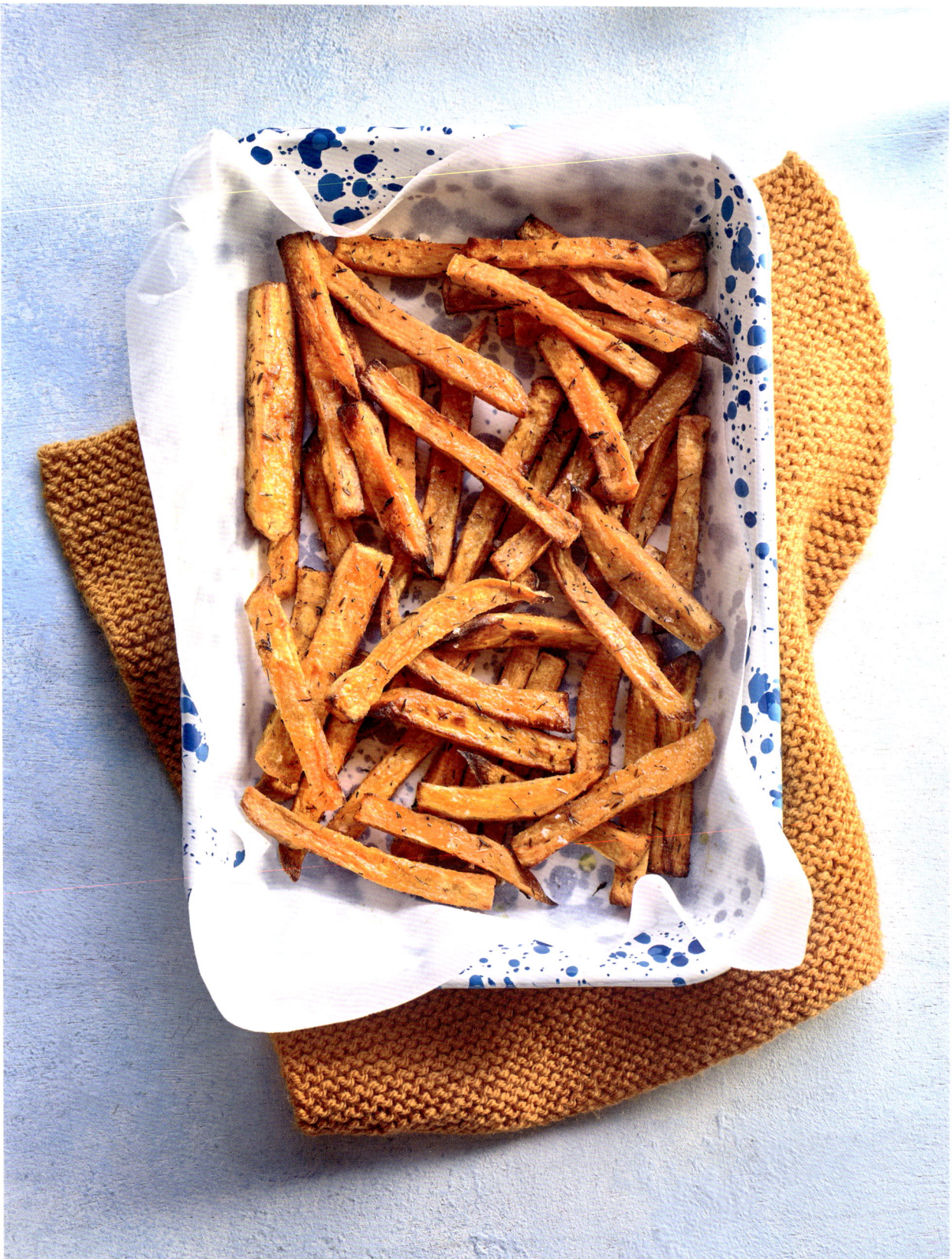

Air Fryer Sweet Potato Chips

These sweet potato chips are just as good as a side dish as they are as a snack. Garlic granules and dried herbs are used here – but there are so many flavour options that would work, such as ground cumin, paprika or Cajun seasoning. Why not experiment with the children to encourage them to try different flavours?

Prep time 5 minutes | **Cook time** 20–25 minutes | **Serves** 2–4

Ingredients
½ tsp garlic granules
½ tsp dried herbs (such as thyme or rosemary)
2 tsp olive oil
2 medium sweet potatoes, peeled and sliced lengthways into
    1cm-wide chips (about 500g prepared weight)

Method
1. In a large bowl, mix the garlic, herbs and olive oil with a pinch of salt and freshly ground black pepper. Add the sweet potato chips and toss until thoroughly coated.
2. Cook in an air fryer at 180°C for 20–25 minutes, until golden and crisp.

You can also cook these in an oven preheated to 180°C/Fan 160°C/Gas 4 for 20–25 minutes, tossing halfway through. Be sure to use a baking tray lined with non-stick baking paper and arrange the chips in a single layer.

Stir-fried Cabbage Two Ways

There is a notorious battle in many households to get children to eat their vegetables. Try not to think of it as a battle, though – just look at it as a process you are going through with them, trying new things. Some will be a success, some won't, and that is okay. Perseverance is key. And there is hidden power in your store cupboard. There are lots of ingredients you can add to vegetables to make them tastier – here we've given two flavour combinations to transform cabbage into something children will love.

Prep time 5 minutes | **Cook time** 5 minutes | **Serves** 4

Ingredients
½ large Savoy or white cabbage
1 tbsp olive oil

For the flavouring
1cm piece of fresh ginger, peeled and finely grated
1 tsp mild curry powder
Squeeze of lemon juice
or
1 garlic clove, finely sliced
1 tbsp soy sauce

Method
1. Discard the tough outer layers of the cabbage and finely shred the remainder.
2. Place the oil in a large wok or non-stick frying pan over a high heat. When hot, add the cabbage and ginger, if using, and stir fry for 3 minutes, until softened. If using garlic, add it now and cook for 1 minute.
3. Depending on your choice of flavouring, either add curry powder and lemon juice to the gingery cabbage, or add soy sauce to the garlicky cabbage, and cook for another 30 seconds.
4. Serve immediately.

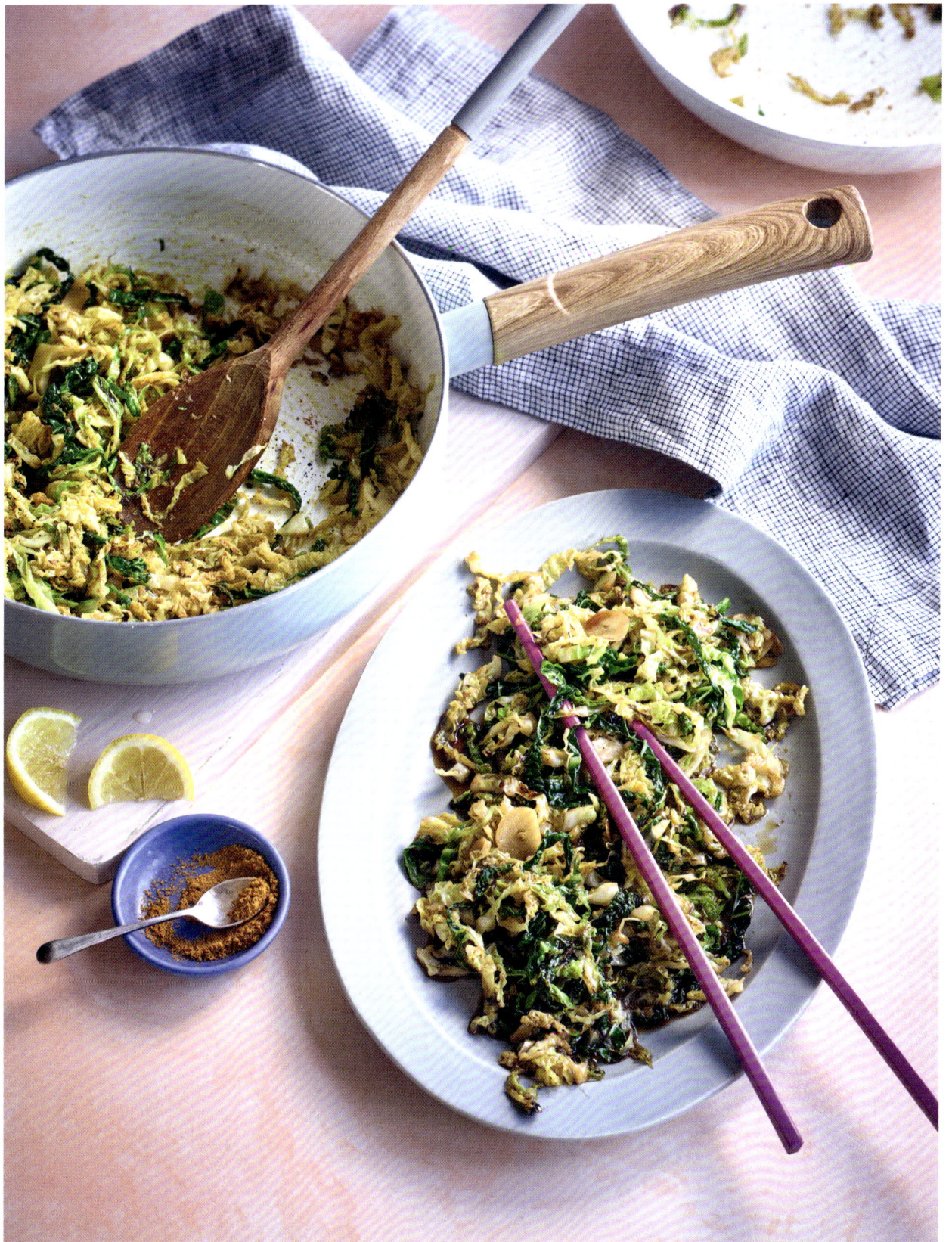

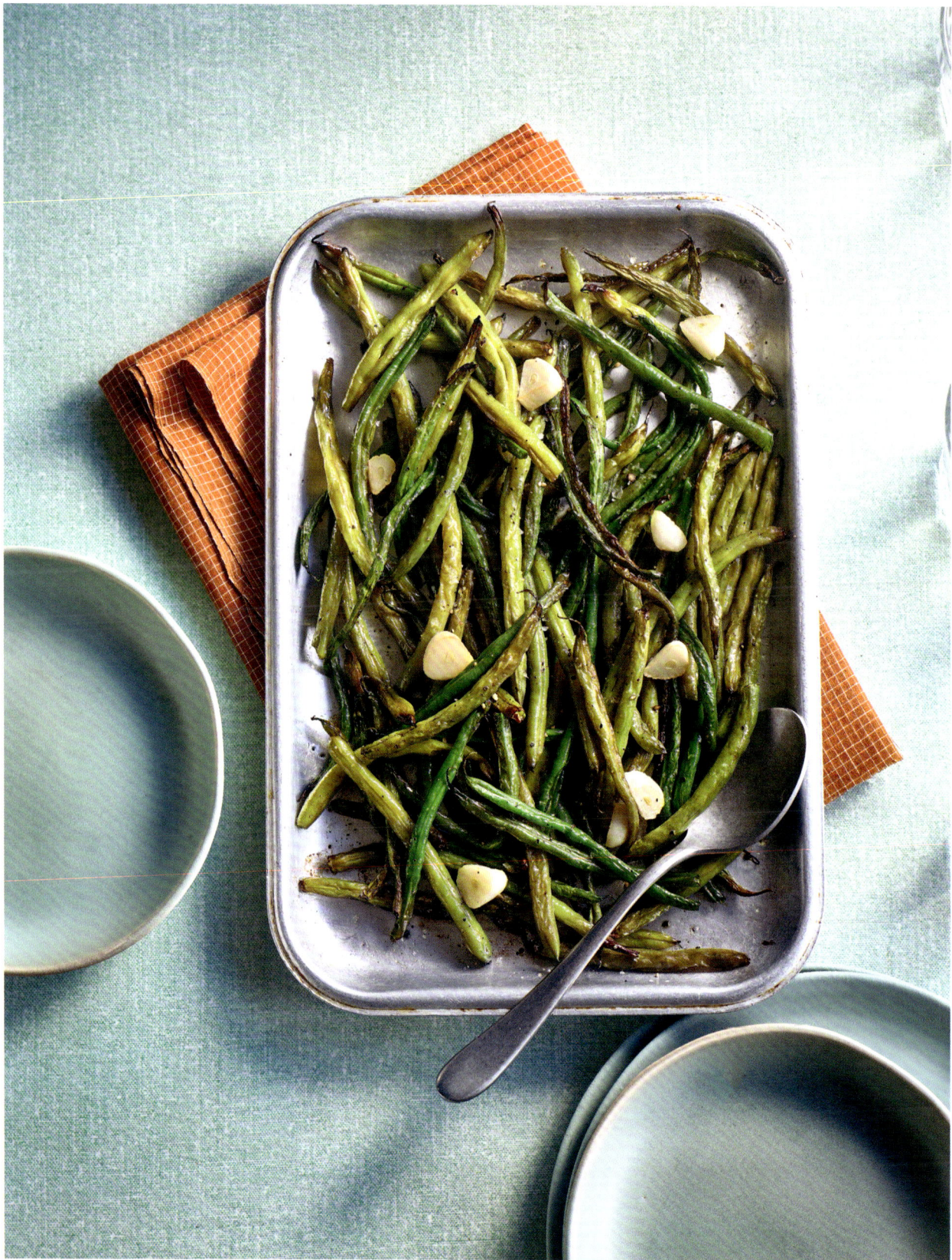

Garlicky Green Beans

These gorgeous, garlicky green beans are so delicious you could eat a whole plate on their own as the French do – drizzled with olive oil and a little butter, if you like. The beans are also super easy to grow in a pot.

Prep time 5 minutes | **Cook time** 15–20 minutes | **Serves** 2

Ingredients
200g green beans, trimmed and halved
3-4 garlic cloves, halved
1-2 tbsp olive oil
15g butter (optional)

Method
1. Preheat the oven to 190°C/Fan 170°C/Gas 5.
2. Place the green beans in a small roasting dish. Scatter the garlic all over and drizzle with 1 tablespoon olive oil. Add the butter, if using, or another tablespoon of oil, and season with a pinch of salt and some freshly ground black pepper. Roast in the preheated oven for 15–20 minutes, tossing halfway through. The beans are ready when they are slightly charred and tender.
3. Remove the chunks of garlic before serving – they are simply there to add flavour.

Mash the leftover roasted garlic with some butter or oil and use to make garlic bread, or add to soups and sauces for extra flavour.

Roasted Cherry Tomatoes with Feta

These sweet and salty tomatoes make a delicious side dish, but will also double up as a pasta sauce. Simply mash the tomatoes with the feta and toss with cooked pasta. The tomatoes are just as delicious without the feta, so don't worry if you don't have any.

Prep time 5 minutes | **Cook time** 25–30 minutes | **Serves** 4

Ingredients
100g feta, crumbled
500g cherry tomatoes, halved if large
1 tsp dried oregano
1 tbsp olive oil

Method
1. Preheat the oven to 200°C/Fan 180°C/Gas 6.
2. Place the feta in the centre of a medium ovenproof dish and tuck the tomatoes snugly all around in a single layer. Sprinkle with the oregano and drizzle with the olive oil. Season with a pinch of salt and some freshly ground black pepper. Roast in the preheated oven for 25–30 minutes, until the tomatoes are bursting open and starting to caramelise, and the feta is melting and golden.
3. Remove from the oven and leave to cool slightly before serving.

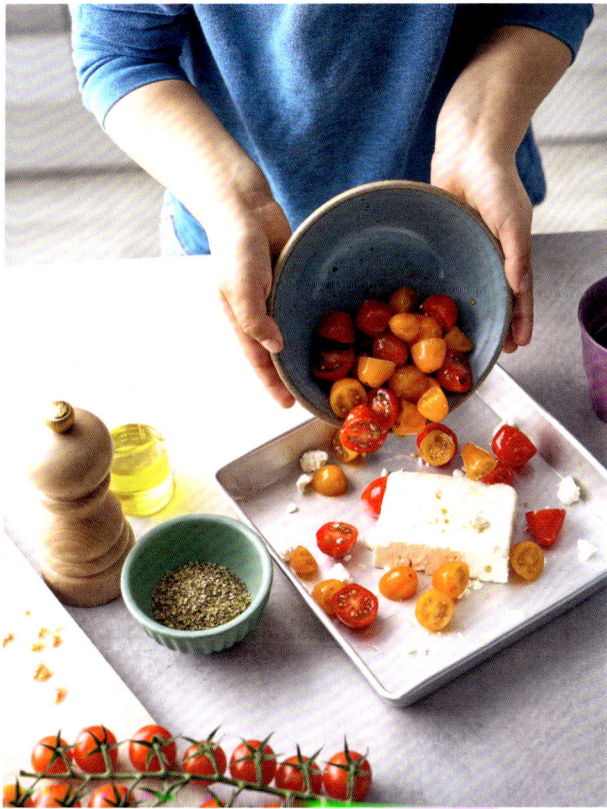
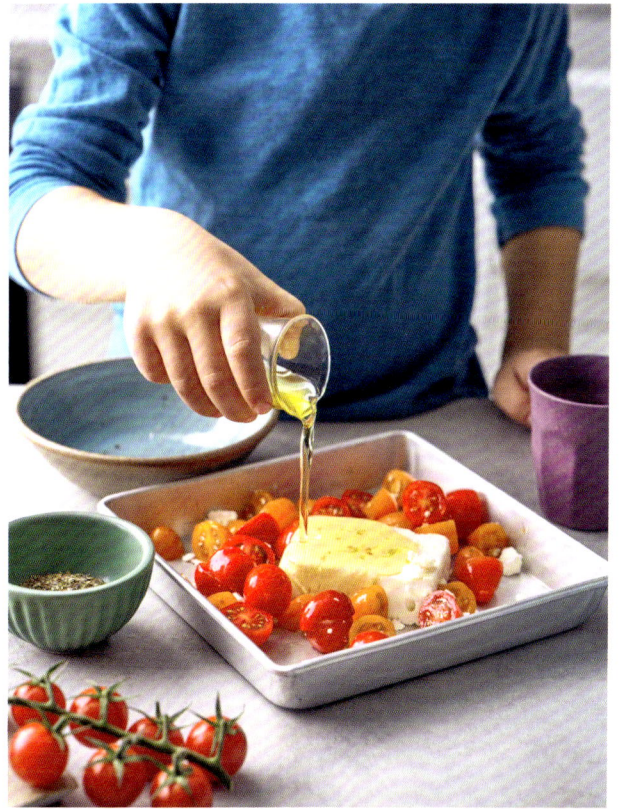
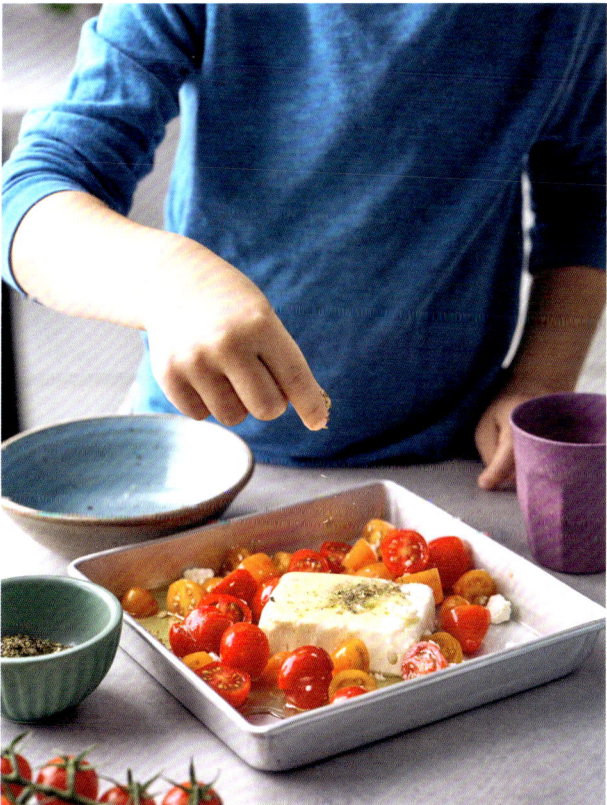
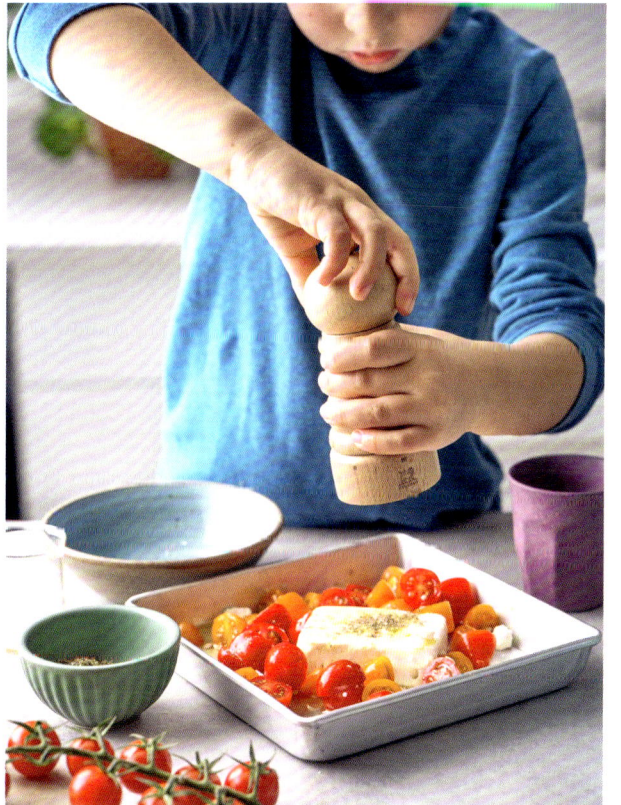

Purple Broccoli with Garlic and Parmesan

There is a logic in saying 'eat a rainbow', because every plant will give your body a different set of beneficial nutrients, from green beans to red tomatoes, purple broccoli and so much more. Try to vary the colour and type of veggies you eat, and encourage children to be curious and adventurous, if you can. I was encouraged to try everything from a young age. If you can't find purple sprouting broccoli, tenderstem (broccolini) would also work well. And if you can't get hold of either, a head of broccoli broken into very small florets is an option, too!

Prep time 5 minutes | **Cook time** 6 minutes | **Serves** 4

Ingredients
2 tbsp olive oil
300g purple sprouting broccoli
2 garlic cloves, finely chopped
Squeeze of lemon
Pinch of chilli flakes (optional)
2 heaped tsp flaked almonds or pumpkin seeds
2 tbsp finely grated Parmesan

Method
1. Heat the olive oil in a large frying pan over a medium heat. Add the broccoli and cook for 3–4 minutes, turning occasionally.
2. When starting to scorch a little, add the garlic, lemon juice, chilli flakes, if using, and the almonds or pumpkin seeds. Cook for a further 1–2 minutes, stirring frequently.
3. Season with a pinch of salt and some freshly ground black pepper and serve topped with the grated Parmesan.

You can swap the Parmesan for 2 chopped anchovy fillets for some added omega-3. Add them with the almonds or seeds.

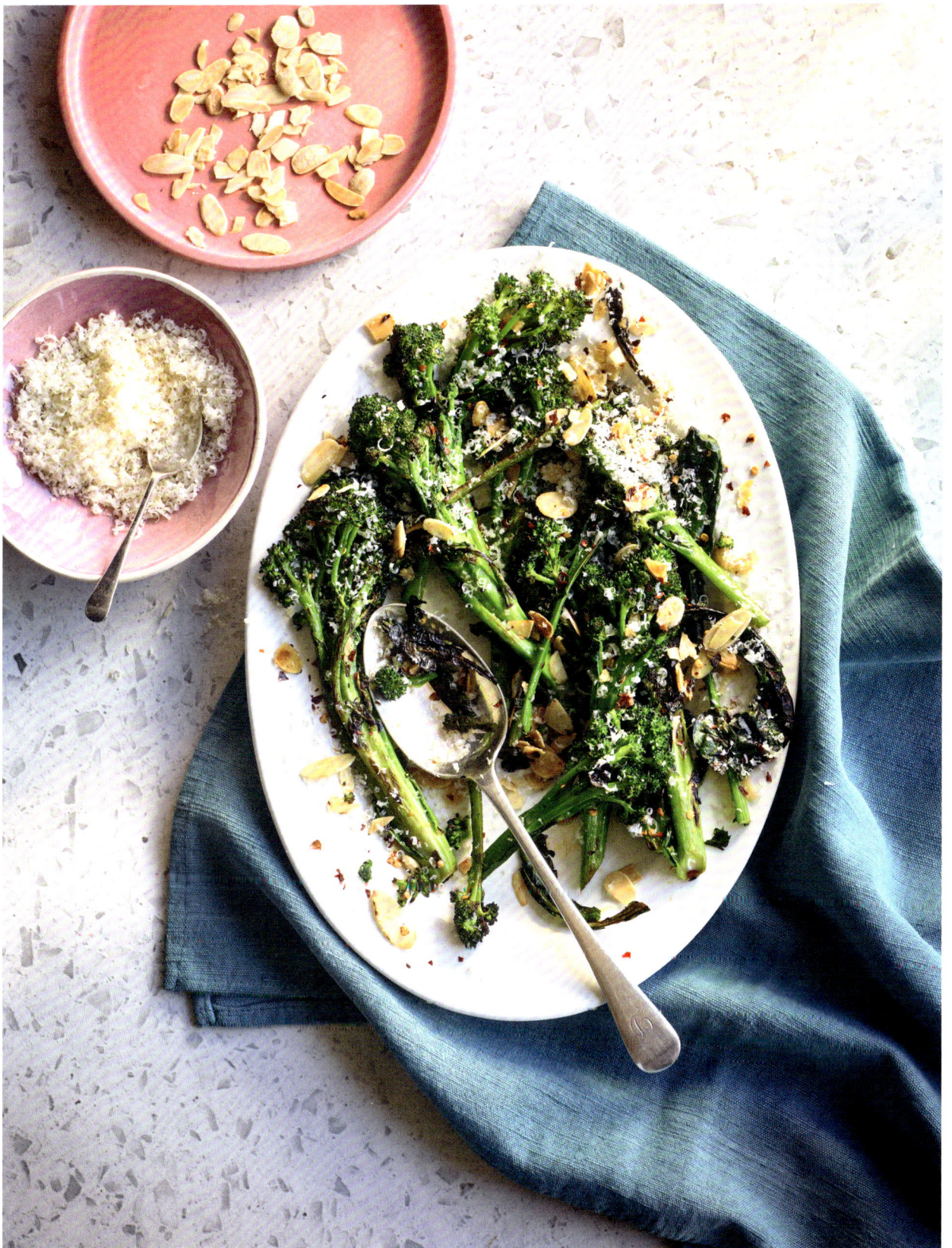

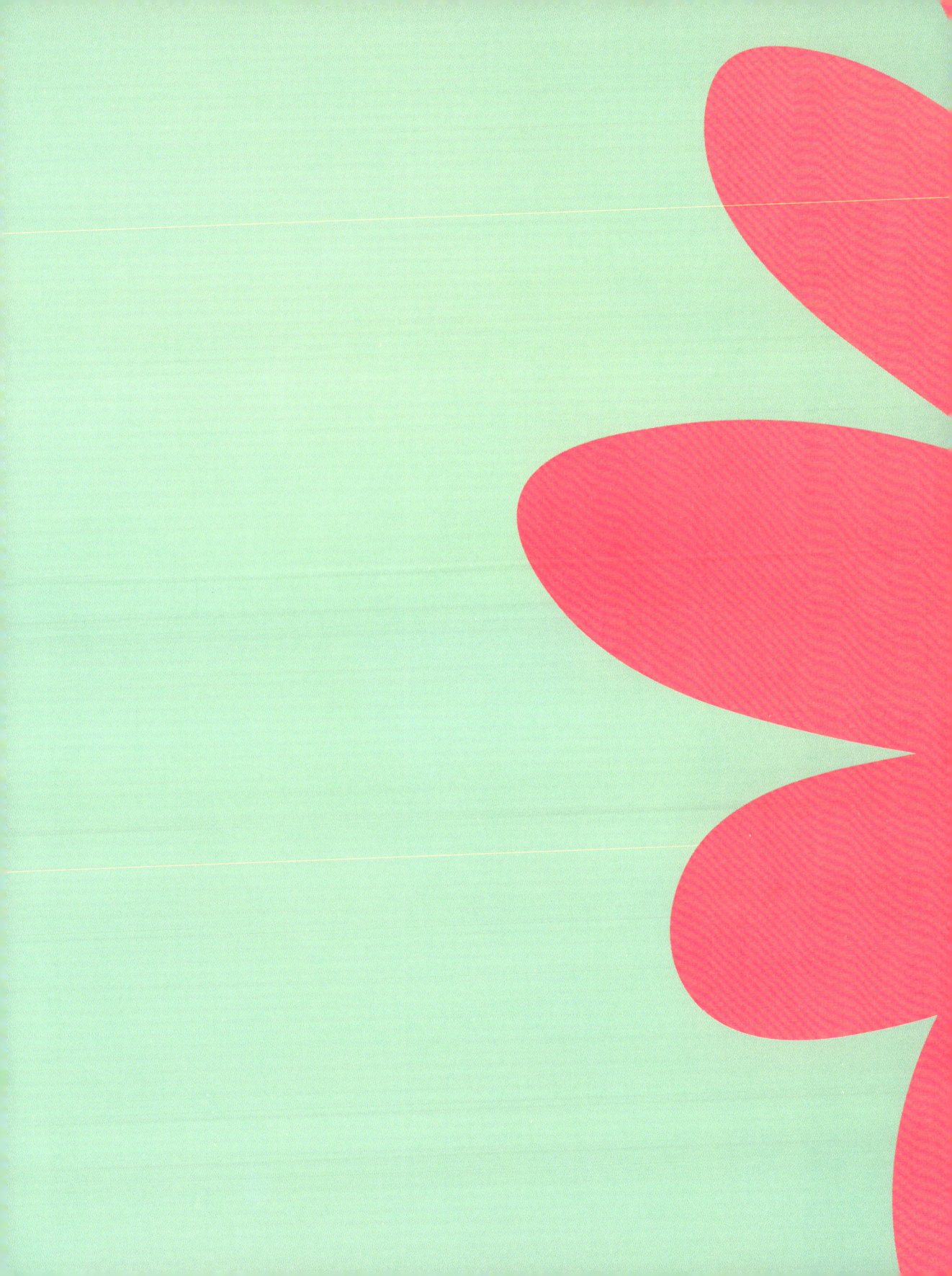

Dips, spreads and sauces

Six Veg Tomato Sauce

I love this marvellous, multi-functional tomato sauce. I remember the days when certain vegetables were seen with suspicion. Here is an easy way to get children to eat a wider variety without disputes! Use it in place of tinned tomatoes in any recipe, toss it with pasta, use it to make the homemade beans on page 86 or serve it on its own as a soup. A food processor is used here to save time on chopping, but cut or grate the veg as you wish.

Prep time 15 minutes | **Cook time** 40 minutes | **Makes** 1.3 litres

Ingredients
1 onion, quartered
2 carrots, quartered
2 celery sticks, trimmed and quartered
4 tbsp olive oil
1 red pepper (capsicum), deseeded and quartered
1 courgette (zucchini), trimmed and quartered
2 garlic cloves, roughly chopped
2 × 400g tins chopped tomatoes
150g Parmesan with the rind attached (optional)

Method
1. Place the onion, carrots and celery in a food processor and blitz until finely chopped.
2. Heat the oil in a large saucepan over a medium heat. Add the onion, carrot and celery, cover and cook for 5 minutes, stirring occasionally.
3. Meanwhile, place the pepper (capsicum) and courgette (zucchini) in the food processor and blitz until finely chopped. Add them to the pan along with the garlic. Cover and cook for 5 minutes.
4. Now, pour in the tinned tomatoes. Fill one of the empty tins with water and add to the pan with the chunk of Parmesan, if using. Stir to combine. Bring to the boil, then reduce the heat, cover and simmer gently for 30 minutes.
5. Discard the Parmesan rind (the rest will have dissolved), remove the pan from the heat and blitz the sauce with a stick blender until smooth. Season to taste with salt and freshly ground black pepper.

The quantities here make a big portion, so freeze what you don't use for another day. It will keep for up to a week in the fridge.

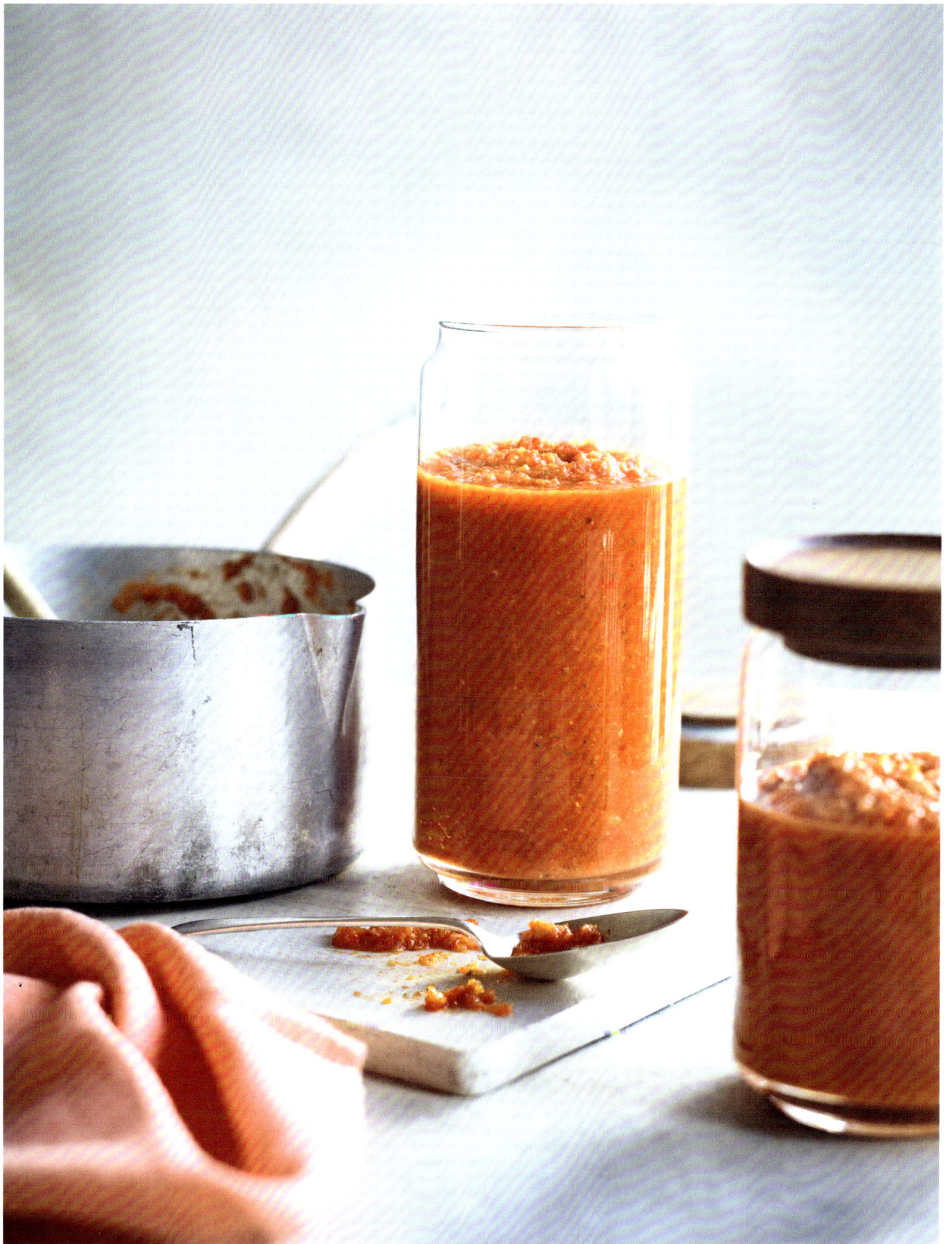

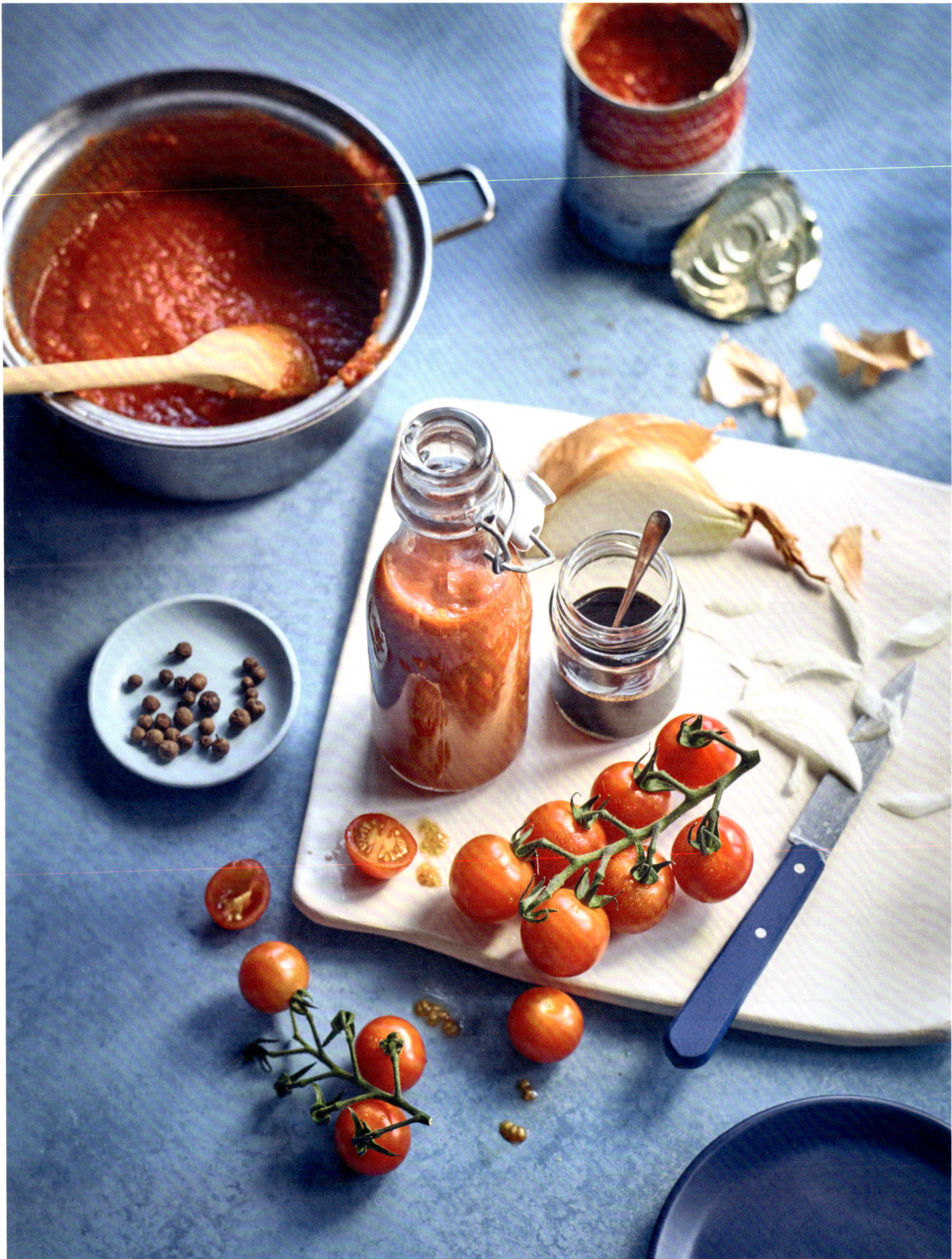

Homemade Tomato Ketchup

Most popular shop-bought tomato ketchups are high in sugars. This version tastes like ketchup, but doesn't contain any added sugar. Get the kids to help prepare it and taste the ingredients.

Prep time 5 minutes | **Cook time** 10 minutes | **Makes** 350ml

Ingredients
2 tbsp olive oil
1 small onion, finely chopped
1 × 400g tin chopped tomatoes
1 tbsp balsamic vinegar
Pinch of allspice (optional)

Method
1. Place the olive oil and onion in a medium saucepan over a low heat. Cover with a lid and cook the onion for 5 minutes, stirring occasionally, until softened.
2. Add the tinned tomatoes, balsamic vinegar and allspice, if using. Increase the heat slightly and simmer for 5 minutes, until thickened. Season with a pinch of salt and some freshly ground black pepper.
3. Use a stick blender to blitz until completely smooth.
4. Transfer to an airtight container and store in the fridge for up to 1 week.

You could also freeze the ketchup in batches. It will keep in the freezer for up to 3 months.

Rainbow Dips

Cucumber in Yoghurt

This is one of my go-to dips. Serve it with crackers, pitta bread or some sliced veg, such as carrots and cucumber. For extra flavour, I add a small, finely grated clove of garlic. It also makes a light and tangy accompaniment for fish, meat and salads. Add other herbs or a pinch of cumin seeds, if serving alongside a curry.

Prep time 10 minutes | **Makes** 130g

Ingredients
¼ cucumber, coarsely grated
3 tbsp full-fat Greek yoghurt
½ tbsp olive oil
3 sprigs of mint, leaves picked and finely chopped

Method
1. In a bowl, mix all the ingredients and season with a pinch of salt and some freshly ground black pepper.
2. Store in the fridge until needed. It will keep for 2–3 days.

Beetroot Dip

Beautiful purple beetroot will help get you closer to that all-important food rainbow – embracing new nutrients with numerous health benefits.

Prep time 5 minutes | **Makes** 260g

Ingredients
3 vacuum-packed cooked beetroot (about 180g)
80g full-fat Greek yoghurt
½ tsp ground cumin

Method
1. Place all the ingredients into a food processor and blitz until smooth.
2. Serve with slices of cucumber, pepper (capsicum) and sticks of carrot.

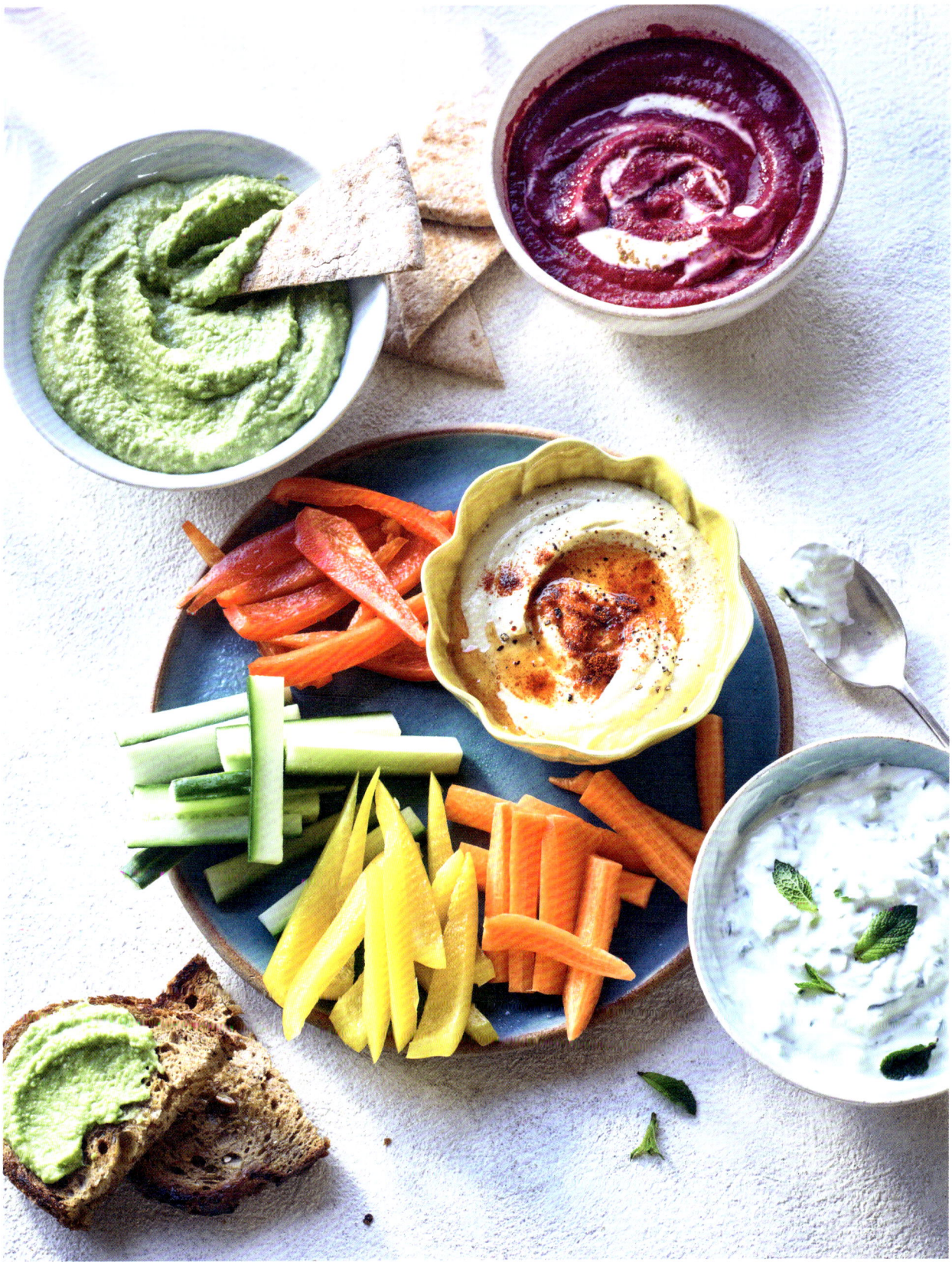

Hummus

The magic of chickpeas – bursting with nutrients and providing a great source of protein and fibre, no wonder hummus is so popular. It's also easy to make at the last moment from your store cupboard. To give it a light and fluffy texture, add a few ice cubes when blitzing.

Prep time 8 minutes | **Makes** 450g

Ingredients

1 × 400g tin chickpeas, drained and rinsed
1–2 garlic cloves, peeled
4 tbsp tahini
5 tbsp olive oil, plus extra to serve
Juice of ½ lemon
Paprika, to garnish (optional)

Method

1. Place the chickpeas, garlic, tahini, olive oil and lemon juice in a tall jug or food processor with 3 ice cubes, a pinch of salt and some freshly ground black pepper. Blitz with a stick blender or the food processor until completely smooth.
2. Serve garnished with a little extra olive oil and some paprika, if you wish. The hummus will keep in the fridge for up to 3 days.

Cheat's Avocado on Toast

When avocados aren't in season, try this cheat's version when you're craving avocado on toast. It's so delicious you'll be making it all year round. Cannellini beans would also work, instead of chickpeas. Try topping it with crumbled feta, cooked diced chorizo or some chilli flakes for heat.

Prep time 8 minutes | **Serves** 4

Ingredients
200g frozen peas, defrosted
1 × 400g tin chickpeas, drained and rinsed
50g pine nuts
1 tbsp full-fat Greek yoghurt or kefir
2 tbsp olive oil, plus extra to drizzle
½ tsp salt
4 large slices of sourdough or wholemeal seeded bread, toasted
2 garlic cloves, peeled

Method
1. Place the peas, chickpeas, pine nuts, yoghurt or kefir, olive oil and salt into a food processor and blitz until smooth. Season with some freshly ground black pepper.
2. Rub the surface of the toast with the garlic cloves, then spread the green dip liberally on top.
3. Drizzle with olive oil to serve.

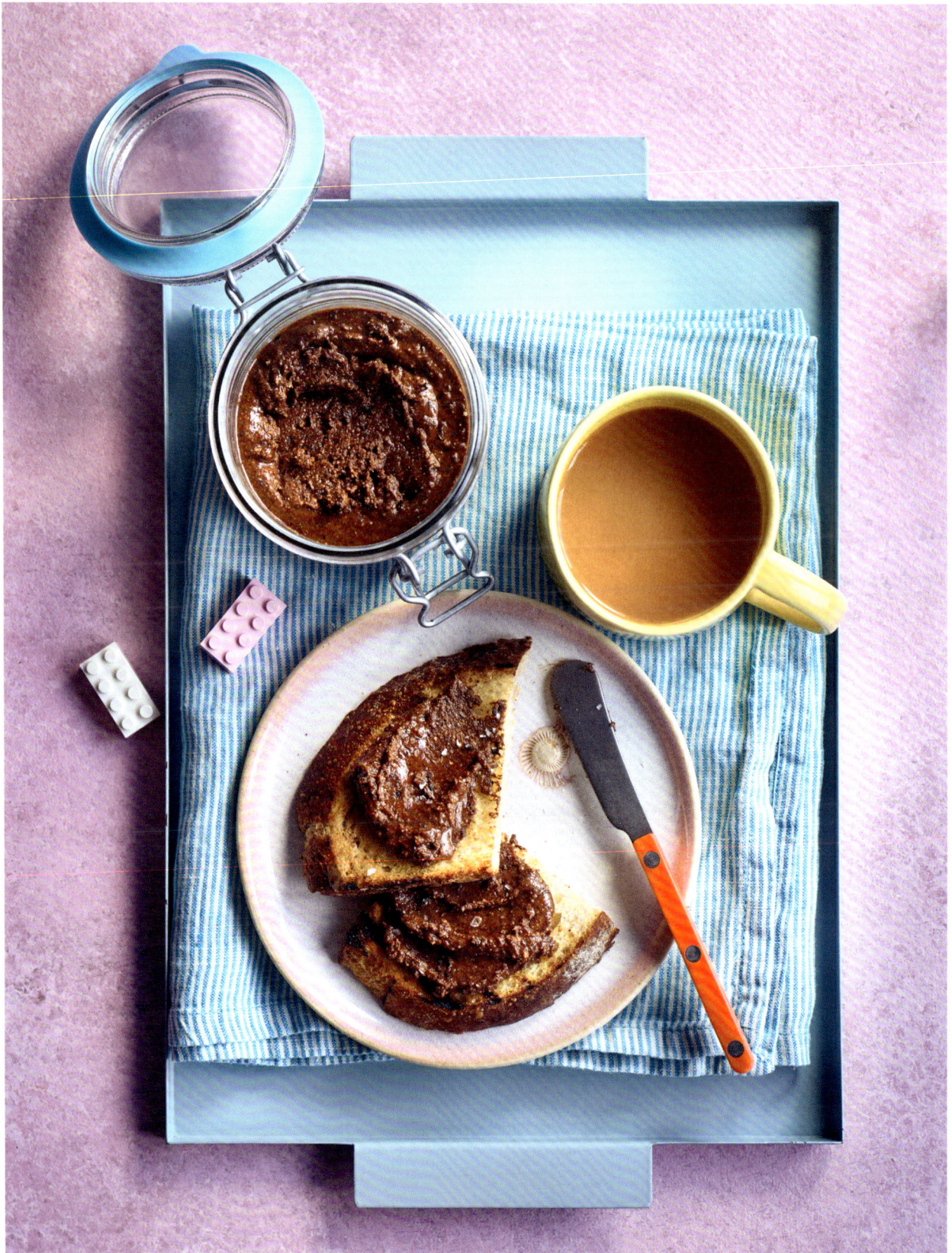

Crunchy Homemade Chocolate Spread

I do like a crunchy chocolate spread, but if you prefer it smooth, blitz the nuts all at once. The team became slightly obsessed with this scrumptious spread, and there are a myriad of nutty variations that you can use to adapt it. Be curious and make your own.

Prep time 5 minutes | **Cook time** 8 minutes | **Makes** 300g

Ingredients
250g blanched hazelnuts
3 tbsp coconut oil, melted (about 45–50g)
50g soft pitted dates, snipped into small pieces
1 tbsp unsweetened cocoa powder
1 tbsp vanilla extract
½ tsp flaky sea salt

Method
1. Preheat the oven to 180°C/Fan 160°C/Gas 4.
2. Place the hazelnuts in a single layer on a baking tray and roast in the preheated oven for 8 minutes, or until golden. Leave to cool slightly.
3. Transfer three-quarters of the nuts to a food processor and blitz for 3–4 minutes, until the mixture resembles nut butter. You will need to scrape the sides down 2 or 3 times.
4. Add the coconut oil, dates, cocoa powder, vanilla and salt. Blitz again until smooth. Add in the reserved nuts and pulse briefly to break them down a little.
5. Transfer to a clean jar with a lid and store at room temperature for up to 2 weeks.

Chia Berry Jam

Yes, you can make jam in 10 minutes! Here we suggest raspberries, but strawberries, redcurrants or other berries work fine, too. However, you may need to adjust the amount of maple syrup. These are perfect for pancakes, to add to puddings or to stir into Greek yoghurt.

Prep time 2 minutes | **Cook time** 7 minutes | **Makes** 220g

Ingredients
200g raspberries (fresh or frozen)
1 tbsp chia seeds
1 tsp maple syrup

Method
1. Place the raspberries in a small saucepan with 70ml water over a medium heat. Bring to a gentle boil. When the berries start to soften, after 1–2 minutes, mash them with a fork.
2. Add the chia seeds and maple syrup, reduce the heat to low and simmer for 5 minutes, until the jam has thickened.
3. Remove from the heat and leave to cool.
4. Transfer to a clean jar with a lid and store in the fridge for up to 1 week.

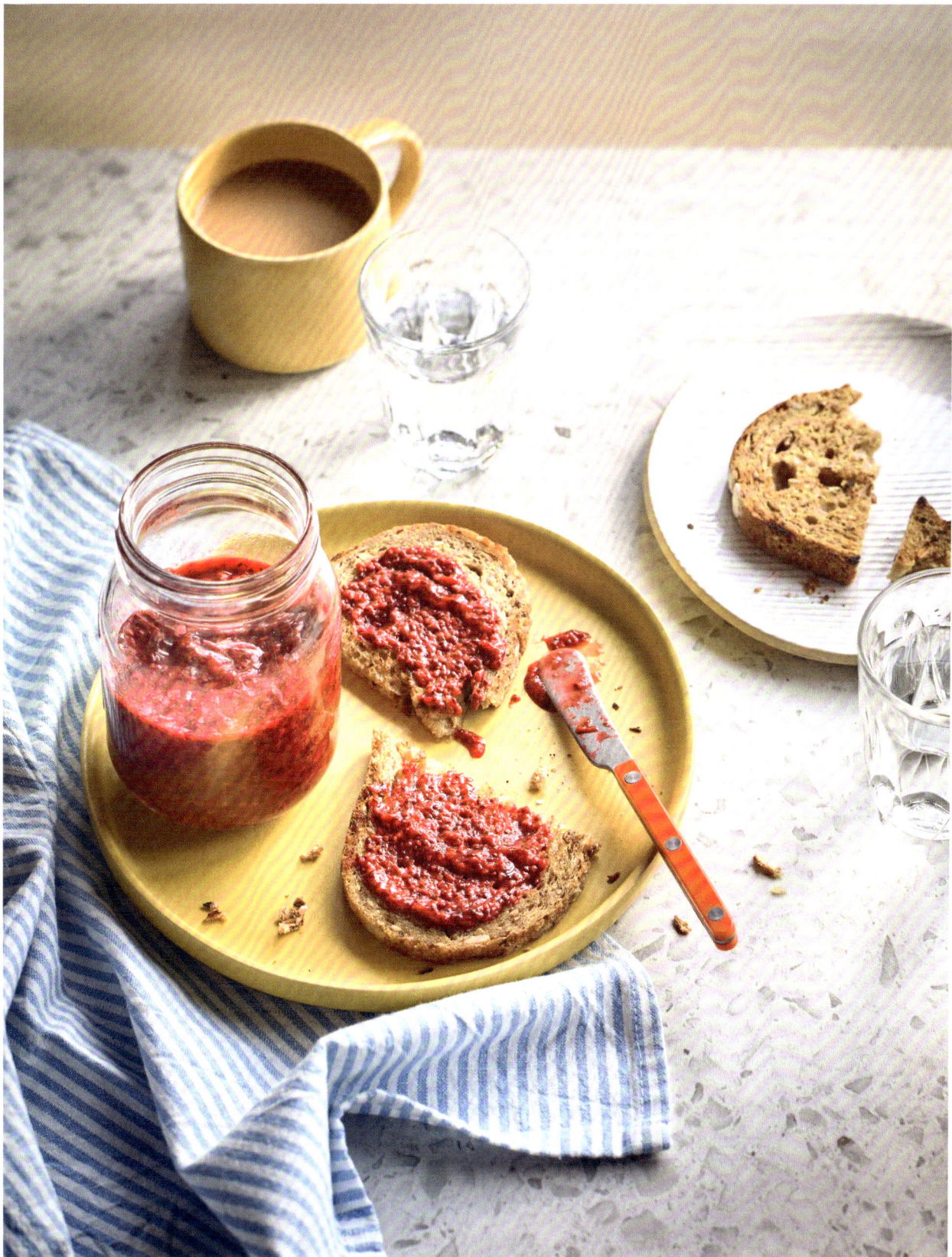

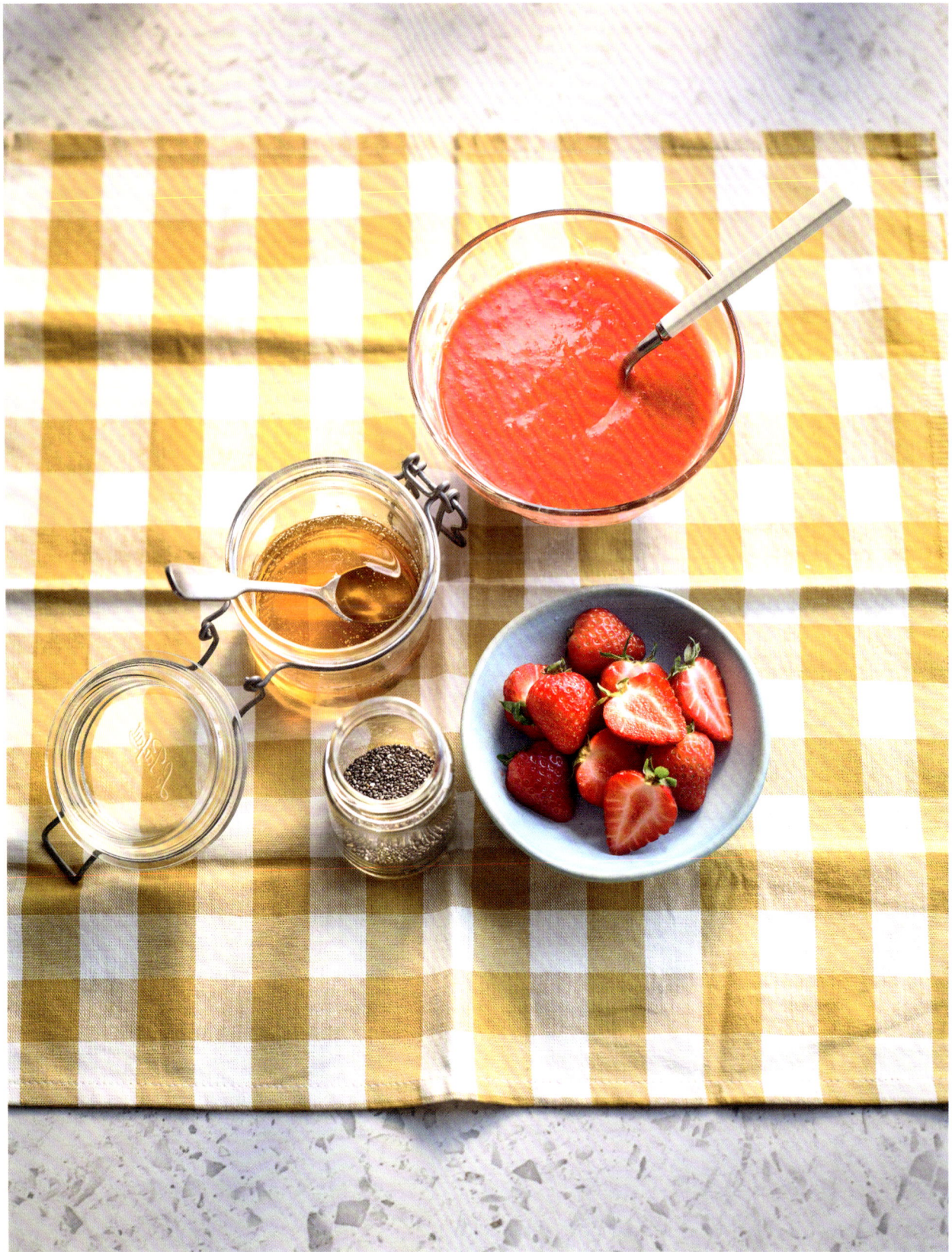

Strawberry Coulis

This delicious coulis is such a great thing to have in the fridge. Children love its intense flavour of strawberry, and it is delicious drizzled on top of, or stirred through, some yoghurt for a quick snack. Swirl it through porridge and scatter with nuts, or serve it with the Sweet Potato Hot Cross Brownies (see page 183).

Prep time 2 minutes | **Cook time** 10 minutes | **Makes** 250g

Ingredients
350g frozen strawberries, defrosted
1 tsp honey
½–1 tsp chia seeds

Method
1. Place the strawberries and honey in a small non-stick saucepan over a low heat. Simmer for 10 minutes, until the strawberries have softened and broken down.
2. Remove from the heat and leave to cool slightly. Blitz with a stick blender until smooth. Stir in the chia seeds (the amount of chia you use will affect the thickness of the coulis).
3. Transfer to a clean jar with a lid and store in the fridge for up to 5 days.

If raspberries are in season, feel free to use them instead.

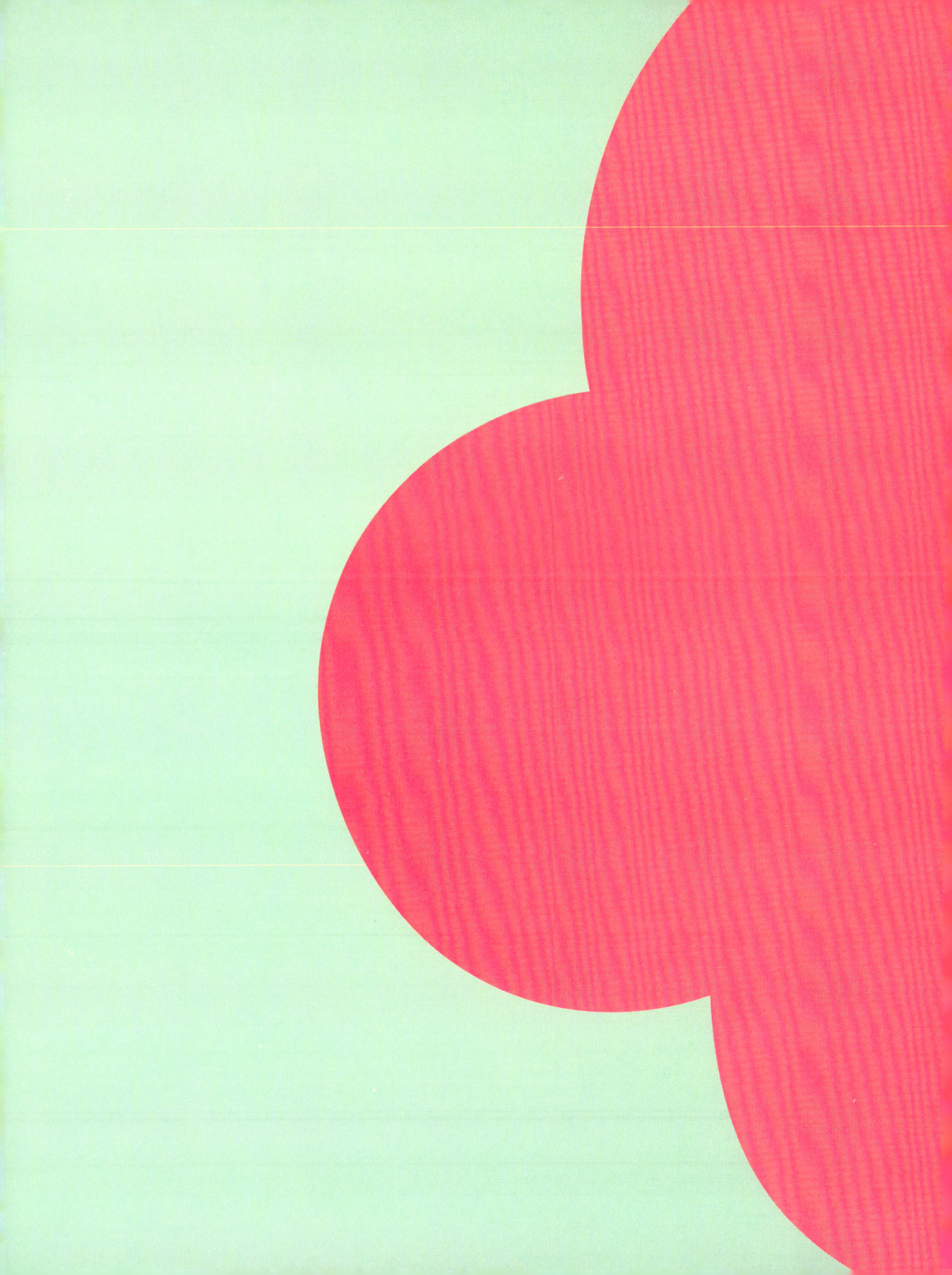

Treats

Oaty Chocolate Cookies

This no-added-sugar recipe is brilliant for using up those over-ripe bananas taking up space in your fruit bowl. I also keep these in the freezer then take one out and pop it in the microwave briefly for a gooey chocolate snack that won't send the blood sugars soaring. They are also a delicious addition to a pudding. I could go on...

Prep time 10 minutes | **Cook time** 12 minutes | **Makes** 10

Ingredients
2 very ripe bananas
1 tsp coconut oil, melted
50g jumbo oats
45g ground almonds
½ tsp ground cinnamon
50g dark chocolate (at least 70% cocoa solids), finely chopped
140g flaked almonds

Method
1. Preheat the oven to 180°C/Fan 160°C/Gas 4 and line a baking tray with non-stick baking paper.
2. Place the bananas in a medium bowl and mash them. Add the remaining ingredients and mix well to combine.
3. Shape the mixture into 10 balls (damp hands will help with this).
4. Place on the prepared baking tray, spaced apart, and press down to flatten slightly. Bake in the preheated oven for 12 minutes, until golden brown.
5. Leave to cool on a wire rack before serving.

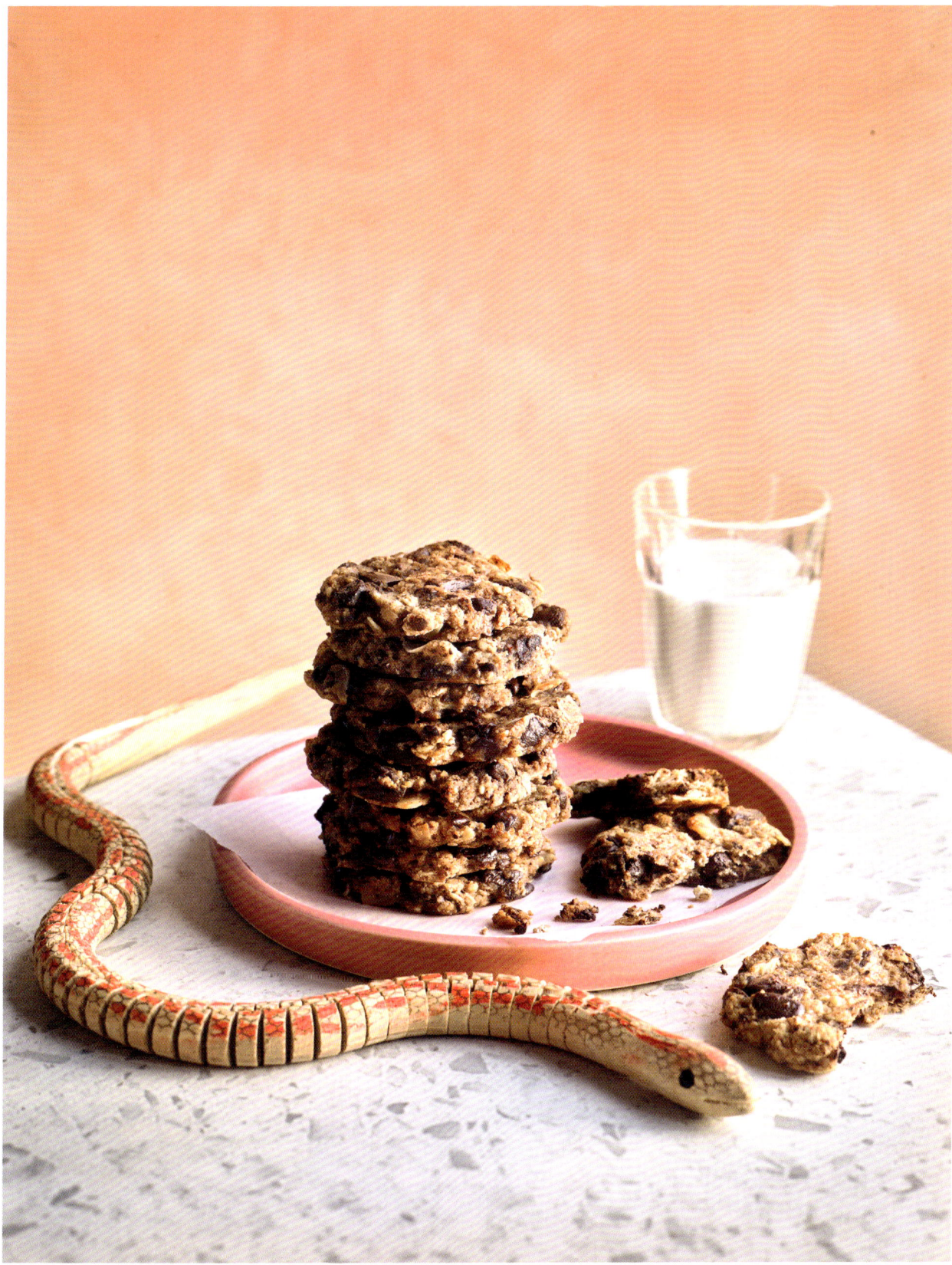

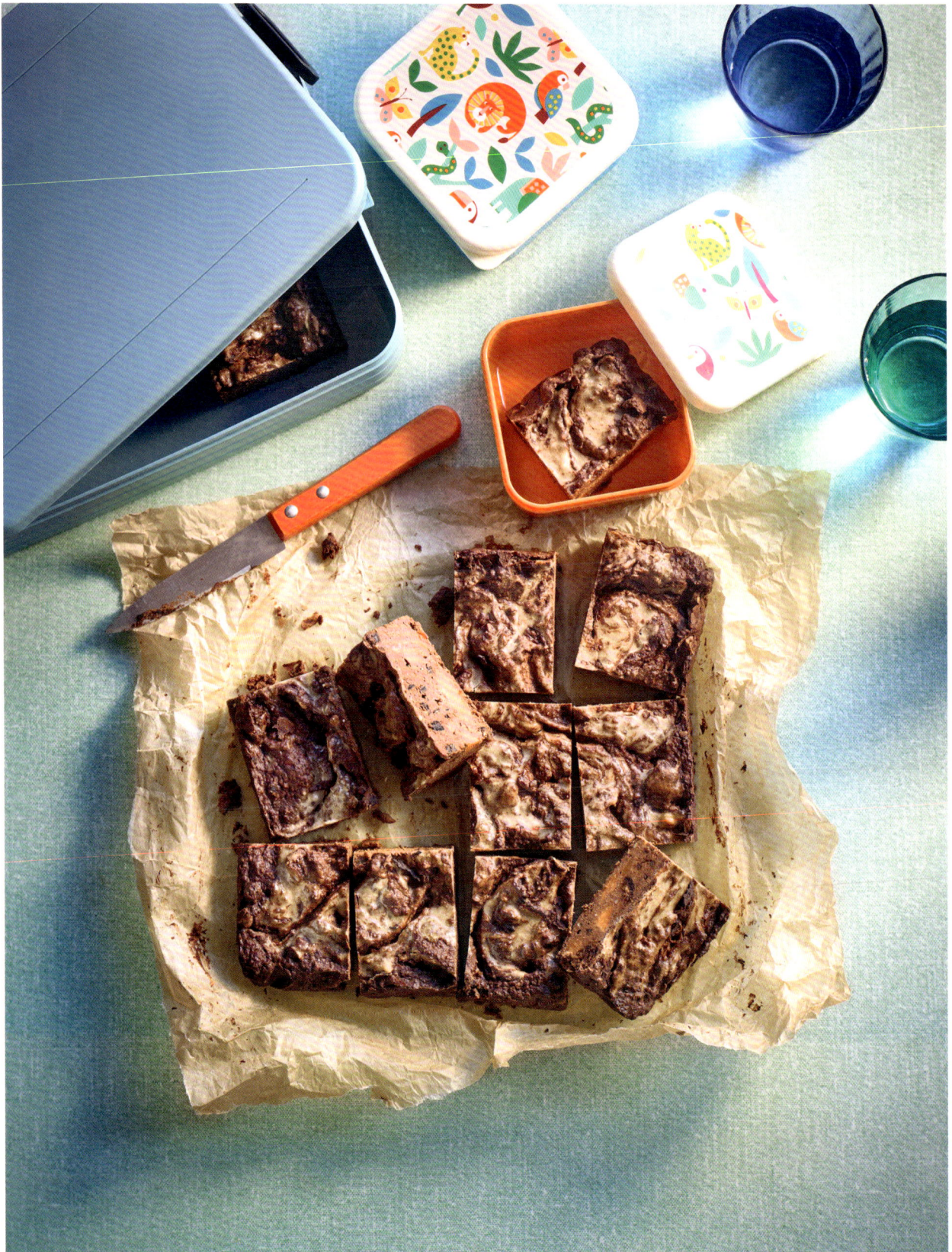

Sweet Potato Hot Cross Brownies

I had fun making this super-healthy version of chocolate brownies, and you'd never guess the main ingredient! These are packed with fibre and nutrients. Children will have fun with the piping, but you can skip the topping, if you wish.

Prep time 10 minutes | **Cook time** 60 minutes | **Makes** 12

Ingredients
275g sweet potatoes (about 2 small; no need to peel), cut into 2cm dice
100g coconut oil, melted
150g dark chocolate (at least 70% cocoa solids), roughly chopped
100g soft pitted dates, finely chopped
75g ground almonds
1 tsp ground cinnamon
1 tsp baking powder
3 medium eggs

For the topping
2 tbsp cornflour or wholemeal spelt flour (or other wholemeal flour)
Juice of ½ lemon
½ tbsp maple syrup

Method
1. Preheat the oven to 180°C/Fan 160°C/Gas 4 and line a 20cm square baking tin with non-stick baking paper.
2. Steam the sweet potatoes over a saucepan of boiling water for 15 minutes. Top up the pan with more boiling water, if necessary.
3. Measure the coconut oil, chocolate and dates into a medium bowl and add the steamed sweet potato. Mash everything together until the potato has broken down and the chocolate is melted.
4. Add the ground almonds, cinnamon, baking powder and eggs and use a stick blender to blitz the ingredients together until combined. Transfer the mixture to the prepared baking tin.
5. In a small bowl, combine the topping ingredients, then pipe or drizzle this over the brownie. Use a fork to marble the topping into the mixture, then bake in the preheated oven for 40–50 minutes, or until a skewer inserted into the centre comes out clean.
6. The brownies are lovely served with a dollop of Greek yoghurt.

Cashew Peanut Bites

These crunchy nuggets are irresistible. Any nut butter will work here. You can even make your own nut butter by blitzing some nuts, if you feel inclined.

Prep time 20 minutes | **Cook time** 15 minutes | **Makes** 16

Ingredients
200g cashew nuts
40g desiccated coconut
½ tsp ground cinnamon
4 tbsp unsweetened crunchy peanut butter
2½ tbsp maple syrup
1 tsp vanilla extract
40g dark chocolate (at least 70% cocoa solids), melted (optional)

Method
1. Preheat the oven to 170°C/Fan 150°C/Gas 3½. Line an 18cm square baking tin with non-stick baking paper.
2. Place three-quarters of the cashew nuts in a food processor and blitz until finely chopped. Add the remaining nuts and pulse a few times until just roughly chopped. Tip into a medium bowl and add the desiccated coconut and cinnamon.
3. In a small saucepan, mix the peanut butter, maple syrup and vanilla extract with 2 tablespoons water. Place over a medium heat and stir for a minute or so, until melted.
4. Pour the peanut butter mixture into the cashews and mix thoroughly until combined to a rough paste. Add ½ tablespoon of hot water, if the mixture is too crumbly. Transfer to the prepared tin and press down firmly using a wooden spoon or spatula. Bake in the preheated oven for 15 minutes, or until golden brown.
5. Remove from the oven and leave to cool.
6. Drizzle the melted chocolate all over, if using, sprinkle with extra cashew nuts, if liked, and place in the fridge to set. Slice into 16 bite-sized squares to serve.

The bites will keep in an airtight container for up to 1 week (they are best stored in the fridge in warmer weather).

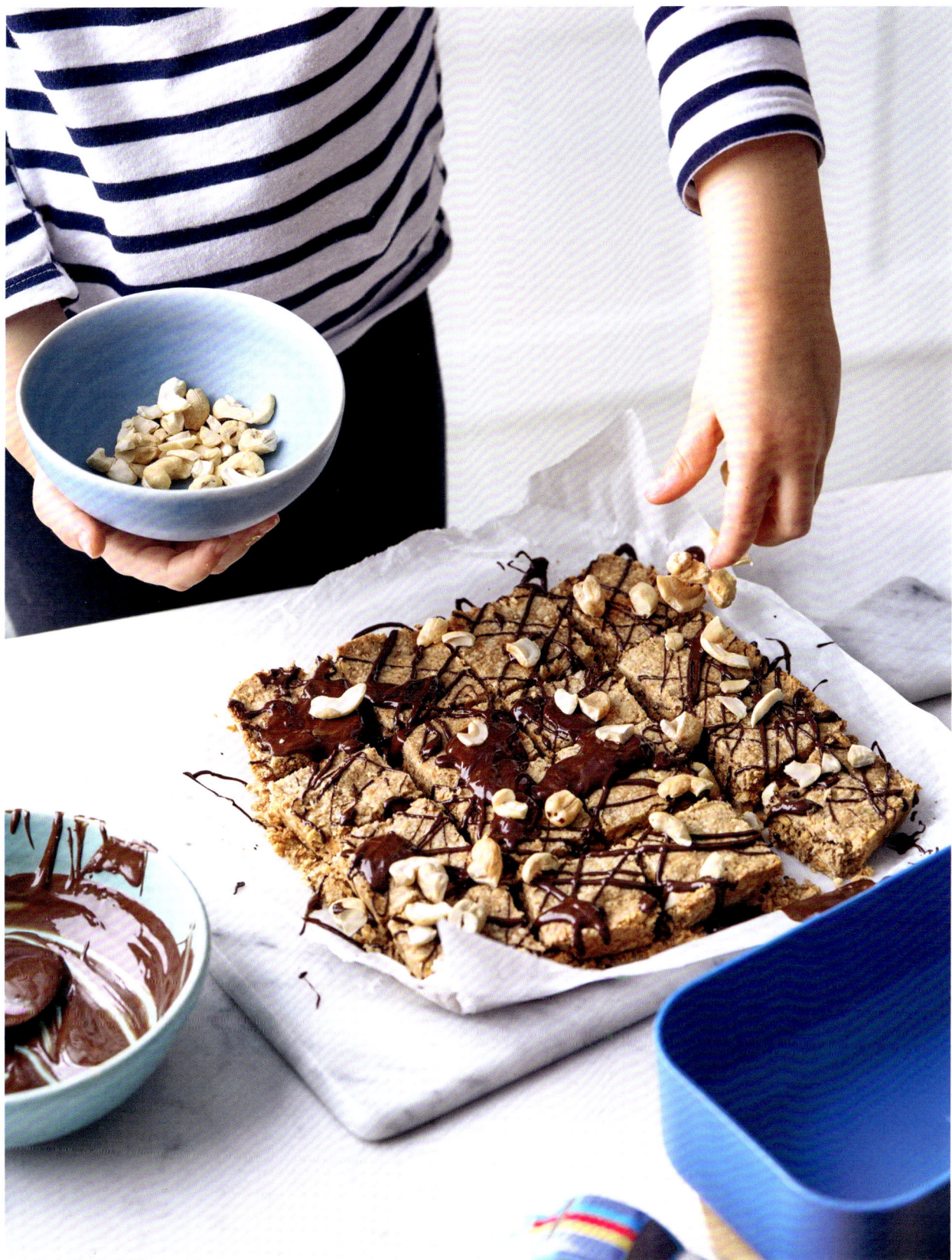

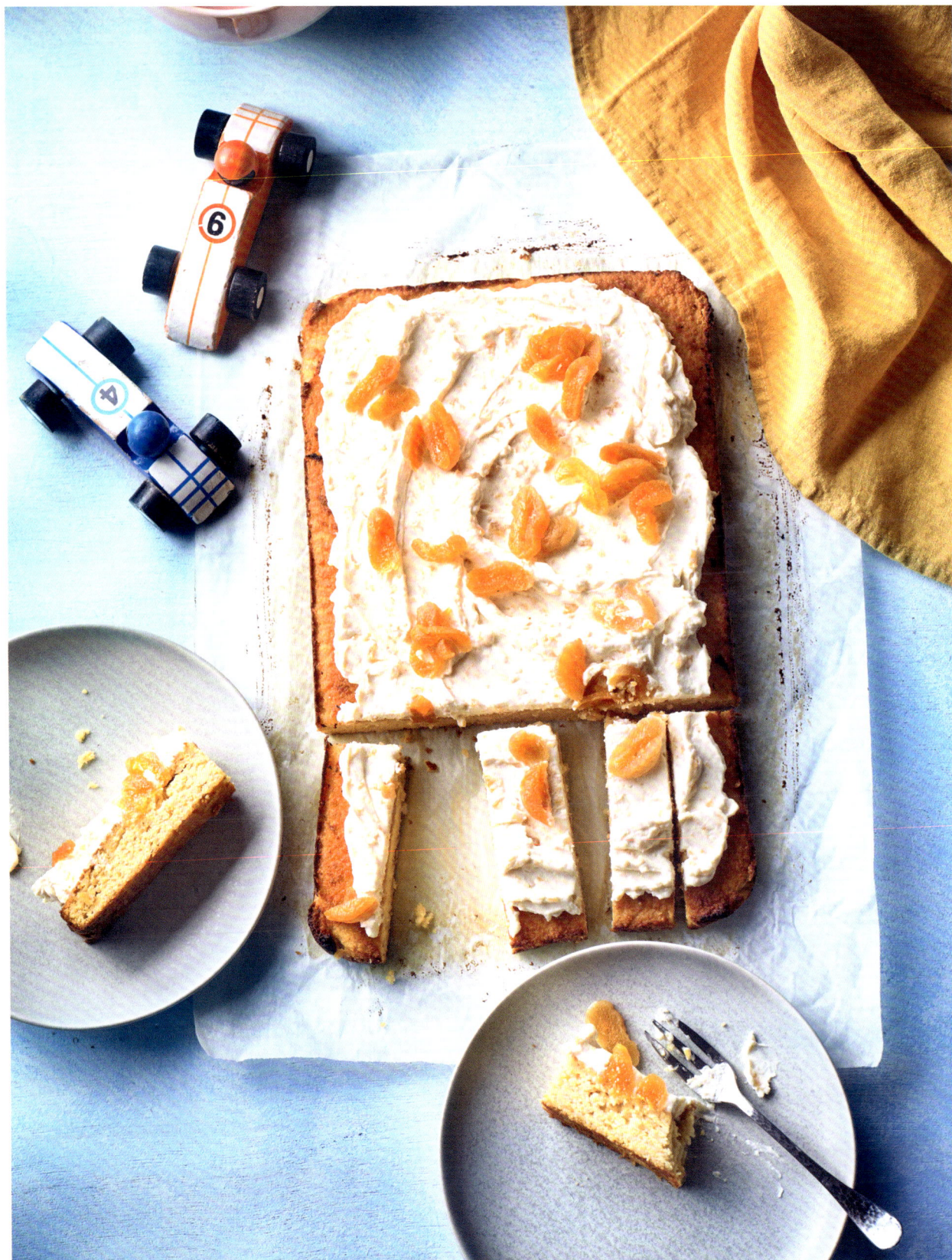

Apricot Traybake

You can't beat a good slice of sponge cake – this one is perfect for parties or birthday celebrations and takes minutes to make. The stem ginger adds sweetness, along with the tinned apricots, which will boost your vitamin intake! The apricot cream cheese frosting is simply delicious.

Prep time 15 minutes | **Cook time** 25 minutes | **Makes** 10–12

Ingredients
1 × 410g tin apricots in juice, drained
75g soft dried apricots, chopped
3 balls of stem ginger, chopped
3 tbsp stem ginger syrup from the jar
2 tsp vanilla extract
2 tbsp coconut oil, melted
3 medium eggs
250g ground almonds
1 tsp baking powder

For the apricot frosting
200g cream cheese
6 soft dried apricots, finely diced
5 tbsp full-fat Greek yoghurt
1 tbsp maple syrup or honey

Method
1. Preheat the oven to 180°C/Fan 160°C/Gas 4 and line an 18 × 28cm baking dish or tin with non-stick baking paper.
2. Blitz the apricots, stem ginger and syrup, vanilla extract, coconut oil and eggs in a medium bowl with a stick blender until smooth. Add a pinch of salt, the ground almonds and baking powder and mix to combine.
3. Pour the mixture into the prepared baking dish or tin and bake for 25 minutes, or until a skewer inserted into the centre comes out clean. Remove from the oven and leave to cool in the tin for about 20 minutes, then lift out by the baking paper and finish cooling on a wire rack.
4. Meanwhile, to make the frosting, place all the ingredients in a bowl or jug and blitz with a stick blender.
5. When the cake is cool, top with the frosting and cut into pieces to serve.

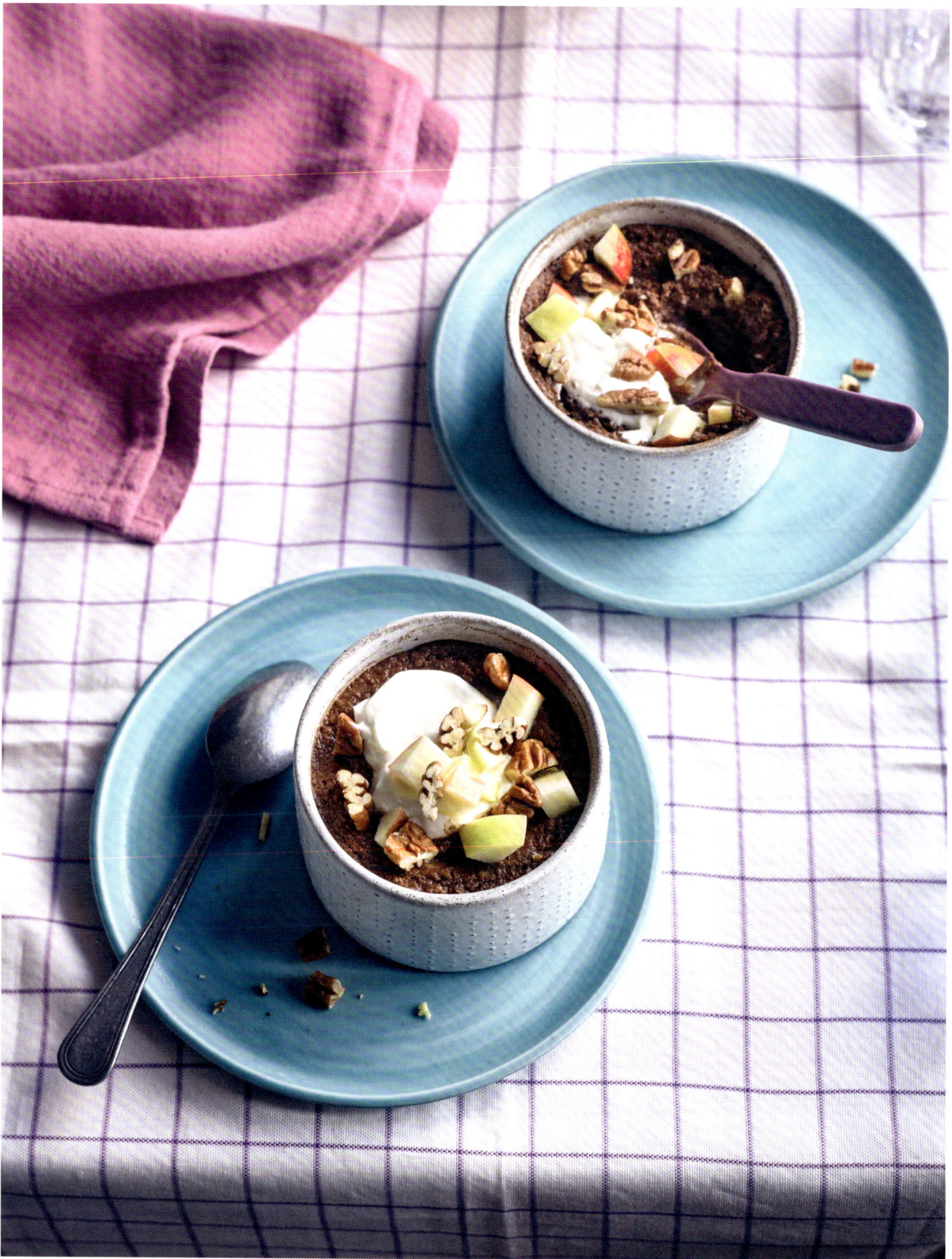

Instant Apple and Chocolate Pudding

In need of instant comfort food? This is a clever and quick recipe which was popular on Instagram and will be on the table in a matter of minutes. Literally. It is delicious topped with chopped nuts, diced apple or Greek yoghurt.

Prep time 3 minutes | **Cook time** 1½–2½ minutes | **Serves** 2

Ingredients
2 small eating apples, cored and roughly chopped (200g prepared weight)
1½ tbsp unsweetened cocoa powder
1 medium egg
1 tsp vanilla extract
1 tsp maple syrup

Method
1. Place all the ingredients in a blender with a pinch of salt and blitz until smooth.
2. Transfer to two heatproof ramekins and microwave on high for 1½–2½ minutes, until firm.
3. Leave to cool slightly before serving topped with chopped nuts, diced apple or some Greek yoghurt.

Carrot Mug Cake

Cakes are getting easier and quicker from conception to the first indulgent bite. Although it is almost 'fast food', this fabulous carrot mug cake is rich in nutrients from the carrot (obviously), orange, dates and ground almonds, which provide protein and fibre – making this healthier fast food! You may find it sweet enough because of the dates, but as an extra treat you could ice it with some Apricot Frosting (see page 187).

Prep time 8 minutes | **Cook time** 1½ minutes | **Serves** 1–2

Ingredients
½ tsp coconut oil, melted
1 medium egg
5 soft pitted dates, finely diced
1 tsp vanilla extract
4 tbsp ground almonds
¼ tsp baking powder
Pinch of ground cinnamon
Zest of ½ orange
1 small carrot, grated

Method
1. Grease a large mug with the coconut oil.
2. Add the remaining ingredients to the mug and mix together vigorously until combined.
3. Microwave on high for 1½ minutes, until risen and firm. Return it to the microwave for 10 second bursts, if necessary, until firm.
4. Serve with Greek yoghurt or crème fraîche.

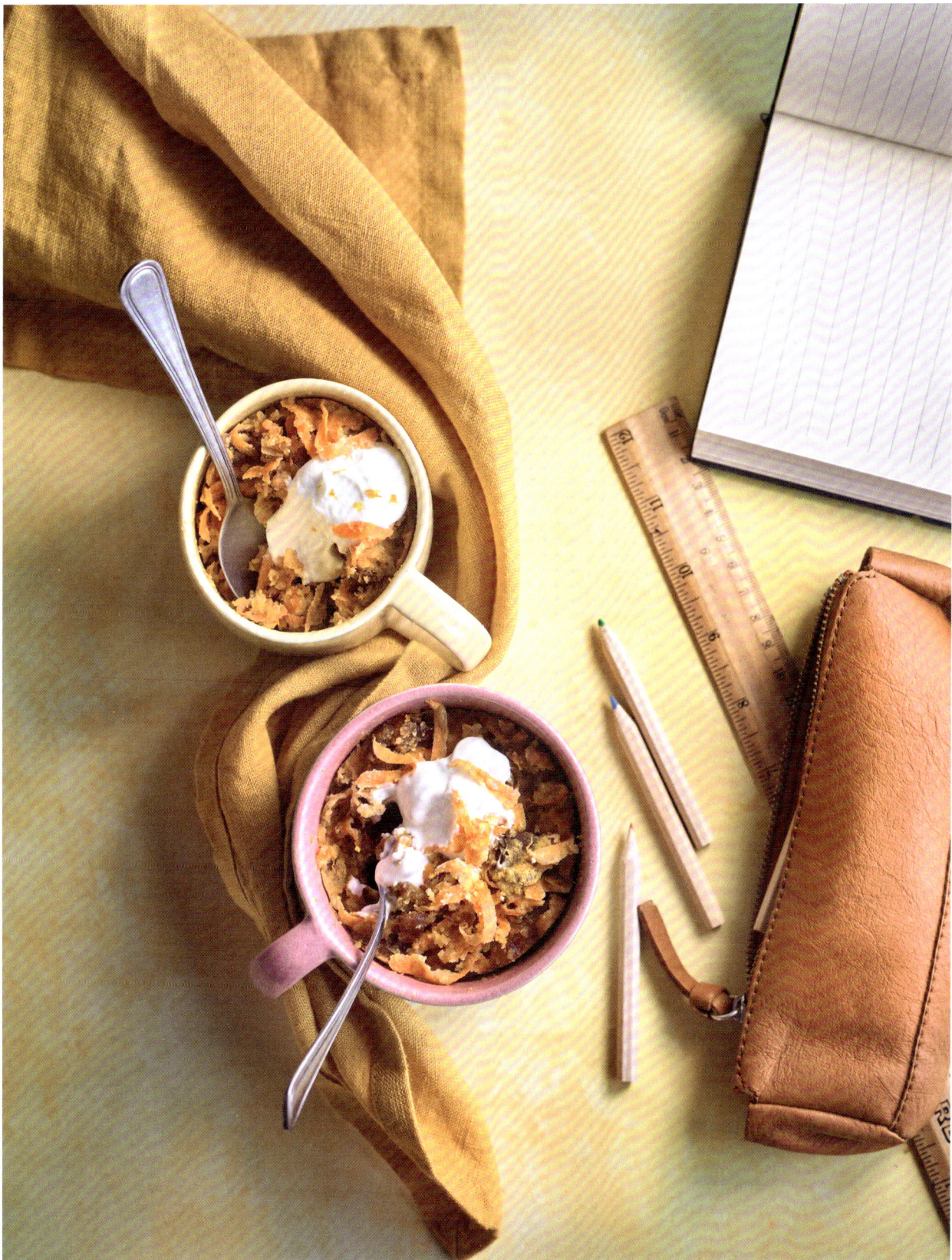

Dairy-free Strawberry Ice Cream

With a wonderful creamy texture, this dairy-free ice cream is surprisingly full of protein and fibre. And, most importantly, it tastes magnificently indulgent.

Prep time 8 minutes, plus soaking and freezing | **Serves** 4–6

Ingredients
100g cashew nuts
1 × 160ml tin coconut cream
250g fresh strawberries
1 ripe banana
1 tbsp maple syrup
100g coconut oil, melted
1½ tbsp vanilla extract
Pinch of flaky sea salt

Method
1. Place the cashew nuts in a large bowl and cover with cold water. Soak for 30 minutes.
2. Drain the nuts and return them to the bowl with all the remaining ingredients and blitz using a stick blender for a few minutes until completely smooth.
3. Transfer to a medium-sized container and freeze for 4–6 hours, or overnight, until firm.
4. Allow the ice cream to sit at room temperature for 10–15 minutes before serving.

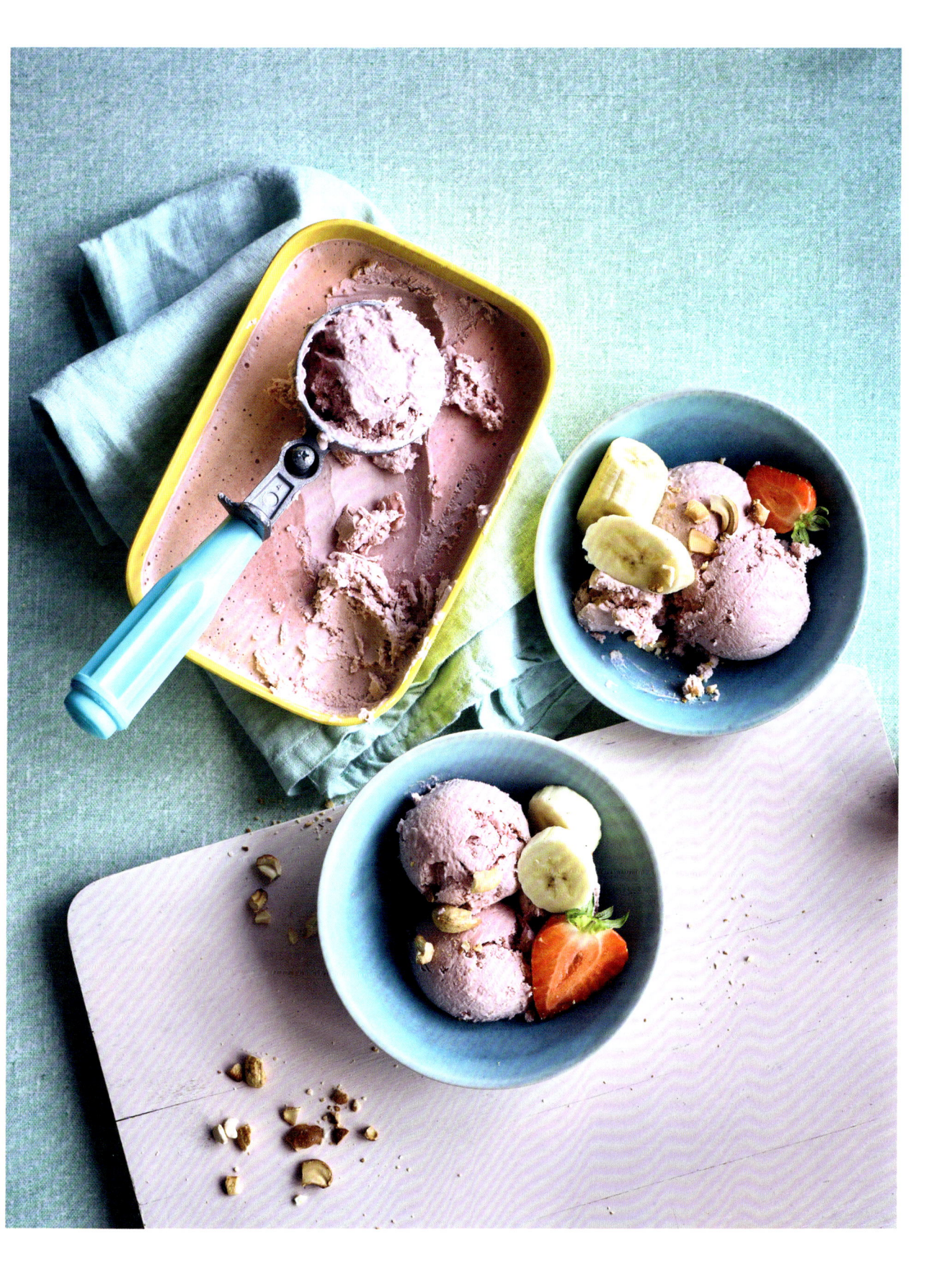

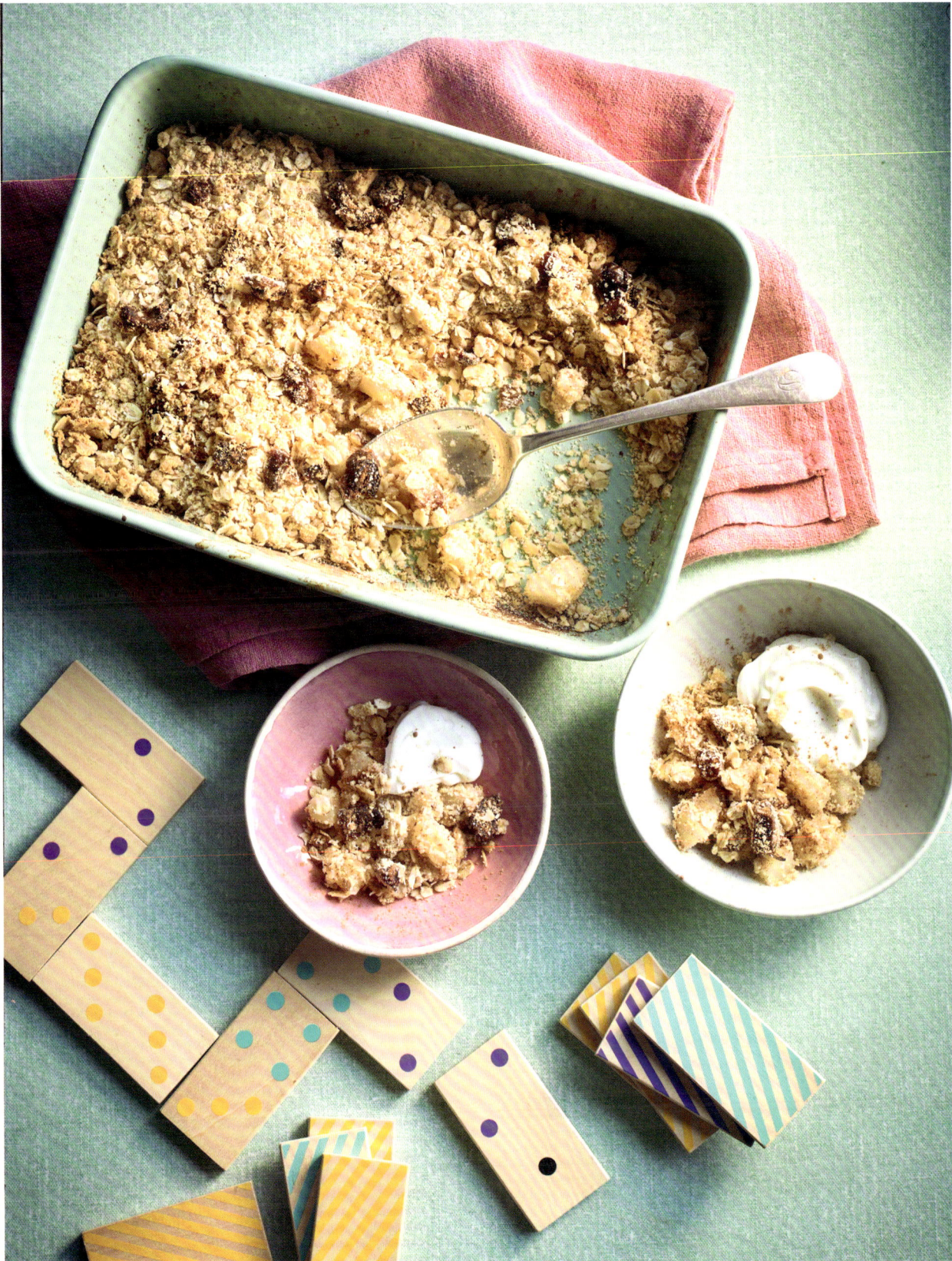

Pear Crumble

Tinned pears are ready to throw in the dish when you need them and are still nutritious. The crumble is full of fruit and fibre with no added sugar. You could add a handful of berries, such as raspberries, strawberries or blackberries, to the pear mixture in the dish for extra colour.

Prep time 15 minutes | **Cook time** 25 minutes | **Serves** 6

Ingredients
50g butter or coconut oil, plus extra for greasing
2 × 410g tins pear halves in juice, drained and roughly diced
1 tsp ground cinnamon
Juice of ½ lemon
100g jumbo or rolled oats
100g ground almonds
50g soft pitted dates, finely chopped

Method
1. Preheat the oven to 180°C/Fan 160°C/Gas 4 and grease a medium baking dish (roughly 20 x 30cm) with some butter or coconut oil.
2. Arrange the pears in the dish, sprinkle over the cinnamon and toss with the lemon juice.
3. In a bowl, mix the oats, ground almonds, dates and a pinch of salt. Using your fingertips, rub in the butter or coconut oil until you have a crumble.
4. Scatter the crumble over the pears and bake in the preheated oven for 25 minutes, until golden and bubbling.
5. This is delicious served with a generous dollop of full-fat Greek yoghurt.

Peach Pudding

So simple and sweetened by peaches, this irresistible pudding is rich in nutrients. And, apart from the egg, you can find all the ingredients in the cupboard.

Prep time 20 minutes | **Cook time** 20–25 minutes | **Serves** 6

Ingredients
50g coconut oil, plus extra for greasing
2 × 410g tins sliced peaches in juice, drained
150g polenta
2 medium eggs
1 tsp baking powder
1 tsp vanilla extract
1 tsp almond essence
1 ball of stem ginger, chopped
2 tbsp stem ginger syrup from the jar
2 tbsp flaked almonds

Method
1. Preheat the oven to 180°C/Fan 160°C/Gas 4 and grease a 20cm square baking dish with a little coconut oil.
2. Set aside 8 peach slices for decoration, then tip the remaining peaches into a medium bowl. Add a pinch of salt and all the other ingredients, except the flaked almonds, and blitz with a stick blender until smooth. You could also do this in a food processor.
3. Pour the peach mixture into the prepared baking dish and level the surface. Decorate the top with the reserved peach slices and flaked almonds, and bake in the preheated oven for 20–25 minutes, until set and browning at the edges.
4. Serve immediately with Greek yoghurt or crème fraîche.

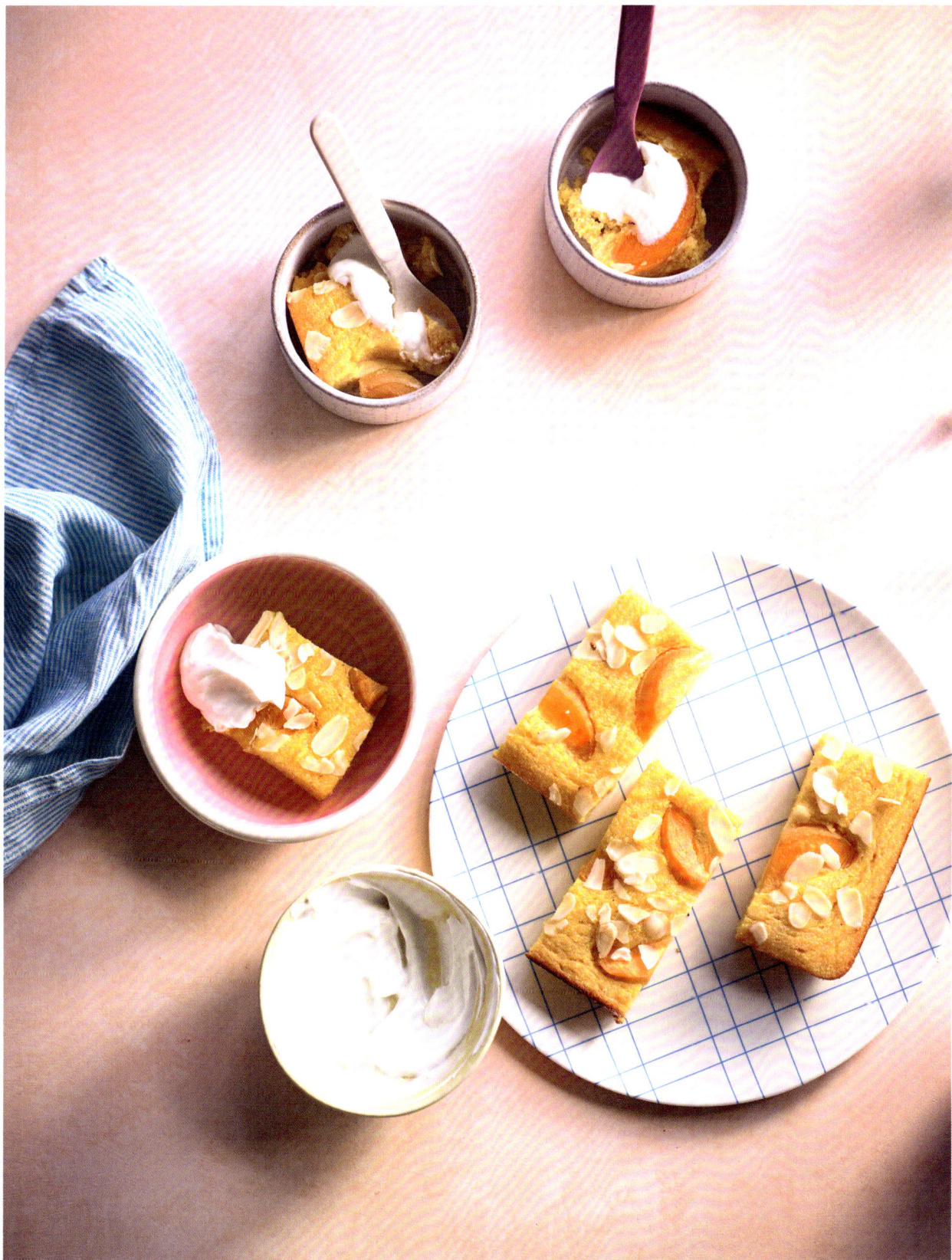

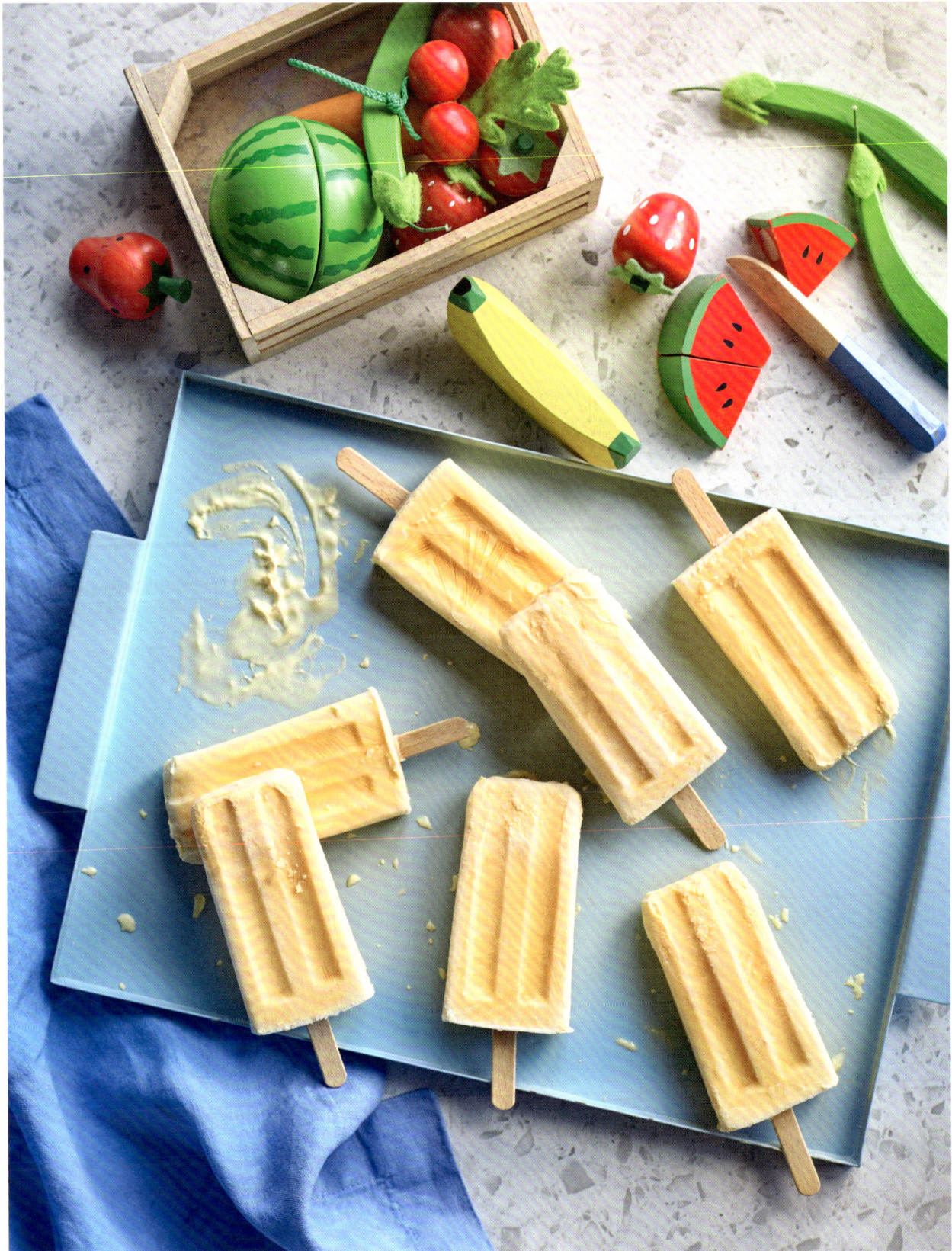

Mango Yoghurt Ice-lollies

You can make these sweet and fruity ice-lollies with a fresh ripe mango, if you prefer, following the same process. Any other fresh or frozen soft fruit will work here, too. You will need 4 ice-lolly moulds and sticks.

Prep time 10 minutes, plus freezing time | **Serves** 4

Ingredients
450g natural yoghurt
2 tbsp maple syrup
100g frozen mango

Method
1. Place the yoghurt, maple syrup and frozen mango in a bowl. Blitz with a stick blender until completely smooth. You could also do this in a food processor.
2. Pour the mixture into 4 ice-lolly moulds and insert a stick into each. There will be some mixture left over – save this for breakfast and serve it with the Make It Together Granola (see page 54).
3. Place the ice-lolly moulds in the freezer for 4–6 hours or overnight, until firm.
4. Remove the ice-lollies from the moulds to serve.

Nutritional analysis per serving

PAGE	RECIPE	KCAL	PROTEIN (G)	SUGAR (G)	FIBRE (G)	CARBS (G)
	BREAKFAST					
50	Strawberry Smoothie	155	6	9.5	3	10
53	Easy Overnight Oats	222	7	15	3	27
54	Make It Together Granola (per 50g)	292	8	8.5	3	32
57	Turbocharged Porridge	295	10	15.5	5	38
58	Strawberry Chia Pots	147	5	10.5	4	11
60	Chocolate Chia Pots with Raspberries	291	10	18.5	7.5	27
63	Apple and Cinnamon Pancakes	115	5	4	3	7
64	Chorizo and Tomato Scrambled Eggs	506	27	7	7	41
67	Eggy Bread with Cheese	288	16.5	1	2.5	15
68	Devilled Eggs (serves 1)	212	15.5	0	0	0
71	Salmon and Egg Muffins	95	8	0.5	0	0.5
	LUNCH					
74	Creamy Pea and Pesto Soup	142	5.5	2.5	2.5	10
77	Lentil and Tomato Soup with Chorizo	211	13.5	6	5	32.5
78	Tuna Sweetcorn Tarts	205	8	1.5	1.5	10
81	Leftover Chicken with Sriracha and Mayo	579	54	3.5	5.5	33.5
81	Hummus, Ham and Cheese	462	27	3	6.5	34.5
82	Green Protein Pots	145	2	1.5	1.5	2
85	Easy Cheats Pizza	300	19.5	2	2	17.5
86	Homemade Beans on Toast	244	10	7	8	37
89	Spinach Wraps with Coronation Chicken (serves 3)	406	42	1	2	6
90	Air Fryer Chicken Satay Skewers	196	21.5	3	2	4.5
93	Traffic Light Protein Pasta Salad	317	31	5	5.5	30
94	Salmon Poke Bowl	510	31.5	4	4	27

PAGE	RECIPE	KCAL	PROTEIN (G)	SUGAR (G)	FIBRE (G)	CARBS (G)
	SNACKS					
98	Cheddar and Almond Biscuits	134	7	0.5	0.5	1
101	Gluten-free Buckwheat Wraps	132	3.5	1.5	0.5	19
102	Seeded Parmesan Crackers	66	5	0	0	0.5
105	Air Fryer Garlic Butter Beans	104	3.5	0.5	4	7.5
106	Beetroot Falafels	50	3	1	1.5	5
109	Protein Power Balls	87	2	7	1.5	8
110	Chocolate Popcorn	70	0.5	6	0.5	9
113	Mixed Spice Instant Muffin	200	6.5	11	4	15.5
114	Spelt Soda Bread (divide figures by number of slices)	2525	74	45	56	300
117	Sticky Nut Clusters	190	8	6	1	8
	DINNER					
120	Parmesan-crusted Fish Nuggets (serves 4)	206	22	0.5	0.5	11
122	Prawn Korma with Broccoli	340	25.5	5.5	4	8.5
125	Sneaky Spag Bol	526	33	10.5	14.5	81
126	Lamb and Harissa Burgers	355	21	2.5	4	27
129	Shepherd's Pie (serves 8)	426	21.5	7.5	5.5	27.5
130	Chicken with Bacon and Peas	524	50	3	3.5	10.5
132	Simple Chicken Stir Fry with Egg Noodles	331	32	9	5.5	26.5
135	Turkey and Quinoa Meatballs (serves 6)	244	21.5	3	2	10.5
137	Sausage Traybake	400	20.5	6	2	9
138	Pea and Pesto Courgetti Spaghetti	511	22	4	7.5	33
141	Dahl with Sweet Potato	358	14	9	7.5	50

PAGE	RECIPE	KCAL	PROTEIN (G)	SUGAR (G)	FIBRE (G)	CARBS (G)
	VEGGIE SIDES					
144	Roasted Pesto and Parmesan Pumpkin	133	4.5	4	2	7
146	Sautéed Smashed Peas	88	3.5	2	3	6
149	Sweetcorn with Butter and Paprika	84	3	2	2	7
150	Baked Spinach with Parmesan	305	12.5	1	1	1.5
153	Air Fryer Sweet Potato Chips (serves 4)	156	2	8	5	30
154	Stir-fried Cabbage Two Ways	55	1.5	4	3	4
157	Garlicky Green Beans	88	3	2	4	4
158	Roasted Cherry Tomatoes with Feta	118	5	4.5	1.5	4.5
160	Purple Broccoli with Garlic and Parmesan	129	6.5	1.5	3	2.5
	DIPS, SPREADS AND SAUCES					
164	Six Veg Tomato Sauce (per 200ml)	235	12	10	3.5	11
167	Homemade Tomato Ketchup (per tbsp)	15	0	1	0	1
168	Cucumber in Yoghurt	62	2	1.5	0.5	1.5
168	Beetroot Dip (per 50g)	36	1.5	3	1	3.5
170	Hummus (per 50g)	170	4.5	0.5	3	5.5
171	Cheat's Avocado on Toast	385	15	3.5	10	35
173	Crunchy Homemade Chocolate Spread (per tbsp)	109	2	1	1	1.5
174	Chia Berry Jam (per 50g)	7	0	0.5	0.5	1
177	Strawberry Coulis (per tbsp)	10	0	1.5	1	1.5
	TREATS					
180	Oaty Chocolate Cookies	174	2.5	6.5	1	11
183	Sweet Potato Hot Cross Brownies	255	5	10	3.5	16.5
184	Cashew Peanut Bites	122	4	3	1.5	4.5
187	Apricot Traybake (serves 12)	255	9	10	1	11
189	Instant Apple and Chocolate Pudding	129	6	13.5	2.5	14.5

PAGE	RECIPE	KCAL	PROTEIN (G)	SUGAR (G)	FIBRE (G)	CARBS (G)
190	Carrot Mug Cake (serves 2)	217	7.5	18	3.5	19
192	Dairy-free Strawberry Ice Cream (serves 6)	350	4.5	8.5	2.5	13
195	Pear Crumble	308	6.5	14.5	3	30
196	Peach Pudding	272	6	15	1.5	33.5
199	Mango Yoghurt Ice-lollies	129	6	17	1	18

Protein top-ups

Protein is essential for the healthy function of our biological systems and it makes meals more filling. The NHS recommends giving your child a minimum of 2 portions of protein from vegetable sources (beans, chickpeas, lentils and tofu) or 1 portion from animal sources (meat, fish and eggs) each day. Here are some simple suggestions of protein top-ups to help you.

Cheese
40g Greek yoghurt (2g)
1 medium boiled egg (7g)
20g Parmesan (7g)
30g Cheddar (7.5g)
50g feta (7.5g)
30g halloumi (6g)
50g soft cheese, such as Brie (10g)

Fish
75g frozen cooked prawns, defrosted (11.5g)
45g tuna, canned in oil (11.5g)
3 drained anchovies in oil (2g)
1 smoked mackerel fillet, around 70g (15g)
2 slices smoked salmon, around 50g in total (11.5g)
100g roasted or poached salmon (24.5g)

Meat
1 tbsp chopped fried bacon, around 7g (1.5g)
1 tbsp diced chorizo, around 10g (2.5g)
2 thin slices ham, around 40g (7g)
1 rasher cooked back bacon, around 20g (5g)

2 slices roast turkey breast, around 50g (17g)
4 slices salami or cured chorizo, around 20g (4g)
75g cooked chicken breast (22.5g)
2 slices roast beef, around 80g (26g)

Vegetarian
40g mushrooms (1g)
2 tsp sesame seeds, around 10g (2g)
Handful of nuts – for example walnuts, pecans
    or hazelnuts – around 10g total weight (2g)
15g flaked almonds (4g)
100g canned beans (7g)
80g cooked edamame beans (9g)
2 tbsp mixed seeds, around 20g (5.4g)
100g tofu (12.5g)
100g cooked lentils (11g)
2 tbsp hummus, around 50g (3.5g)
100g cooked quinoa (6g)

Metric/imperial conversions

Weight

15g .... ½oz
20g .... ¾oz
25g/30g 1oz
35g 1¼oz
40g/45g 1½oz
50g 1¾oz
55g 2oz
60g 2¼oz
65g 2⅓oz
70g 2½oz
75g 2⅔oz
80g 2¾oz
85g 3oz
90g 3¼oz
100g 3½oz
110g 3¾oz
125g 4½oz
150g 5⅓oz
160g 5⅔oz
170g 6oz
175g 6¼oz
200g 7oz
225g 8oz
230g 8¼oz
250g 9oz
275g 9¾oz
300g 10½oz
325g 11½oz
350g 12oz
375g 13oz
400g 14oz
410g 14½oz
450g 1lb
500g 1lb 2oz
650g 1lb 7oz

Volume

50ml .... 1¾fl oz
60ml .... 2fl oz
70ml .... 2½fl oz
75ml .... 2⅔fl oz
100ml .... 3½fl oz
125ml .... 4fl oz
150ml .... 5fl oz (¼ pint)
160ml .... 5½fl oz
175ml .... 6fl oz
200ml .... 7fl oz (⅓ pint)
225ml .... 8fl oz
250ml .... 9fl oz
300ml .... 10fl oz
           (½ pint)
350ml .... 12fl oz
400ml .... 14fl oz
450ml .... 15fl oz
           (¾ pint)
500ml .... 18fl oz
600ml .... 20fl oz (1 pint)
900ml .... 31⅔fl oz
           (1½ pints)

Measurements

1cm .... ½in
2cm .... ¾in
2.5cm 1in
3cm 1¼in
5cm 2in
7.5cm 3in
9cm 3½in
10cm 4in
13cm 5¼in
15cm 6in
18cm 7in
20cm 8in
25cm 10in
28cm 11in

Index

UK/US terms

Aubergine .... eggplant
Baby gem lettuce .... little gem lettuce
Baking paper .... parchment paper
Baking tray .... baking sheet
Beef mince .... ground beef
Beetroot .... beets
Brown sauce .... Heinz 57 or A1 Steak Sauce
Celery sticks .... celery stalks
Cornflour .... corn starch
Courgette .... zucchini
Dark chocolate .... semi-sweet chocolate
Dried chilli flakes .... red pepper flakes
Flaxseed .... linseed
Full-fat milk .... whole milk
Hazelnut .... filbert
Lamb mince .... ground lamb

Pak choi .... bok choy
Passata .... tomato puree
Pepper (capsicum) .... bell pepper
Plain flour .... all-purpose flour
Polenta .... corn meal
Prawns .... shrimp
Pumpkin seeds .... pepitas
Stem ginger .... candied ginger
Stock cube .... bouillon cube
Tin .... pan
Tinned .... canned
Turkey thigh mince .... ground turkey
Whisk .... beat
Wholegrain/wholemeal .... wholewheat
Yoghurt .... yogurt
Zest .... rind

Acknowledgements

Very special thanks to agent Sophie Laurimore. Thanks, also, to Jo Morrell, for your calm, wise judgement and for making it all come together.

Thank you to brilliant food writer Kathryn Bruton, and special thanks to your girls for their recipe testing and wise suggestions. Thank you, also, to Caroline Barton, for helping with the recipe testing and for sharing your nutritional expertise.

Thank you to Yasia Williams, for your joyful design and flexibility, and Lizzie Ballantyne, for your fabulous design input. Thank you to Leanne Bryan, for your excellent editorial input and hard work, and to Jo Roberts-Miller – as calm, efficient and effective as ever. Thanks to Katherine Hockley for putting it all together so well.

Thanks to Kate Whitaker, for the lively and charming images, to Becks Wilkinson (you really made the food pop!) and to Hannah Wilkinson, for the fun and family-friendly tone. Thank you, also, to all the parents and children who volunteered to model in the photographs.